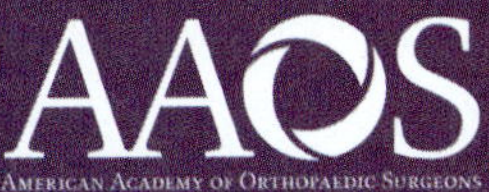

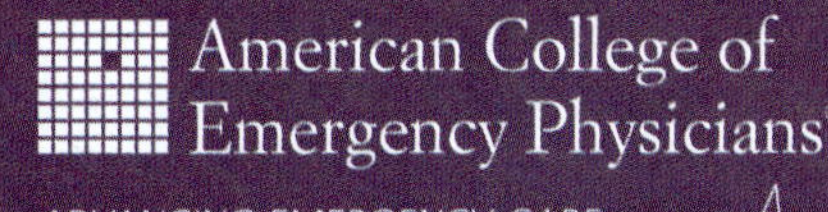

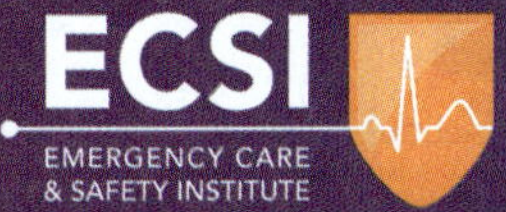

CPR and AED

NINTH EDITION

Authors

Alton L. Thygerson, *EdD, FAWM*
Steven M. Thygerson, *PhD, MSPH, CIH*
Justin S. Thygerson, *PhD, CSP*

Medical Editors

Alfonso Mejia, *MD, MPH, FAAOS*
Nicholas Cozzi, *MD, MBA, FACEP*

Series Editor

Bob Elling, *MPA, EMT-P*

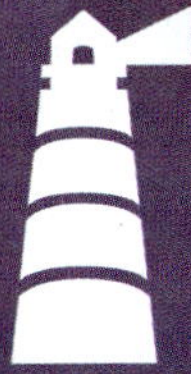

JONES & BARTLETT
LEARNING

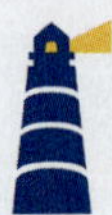

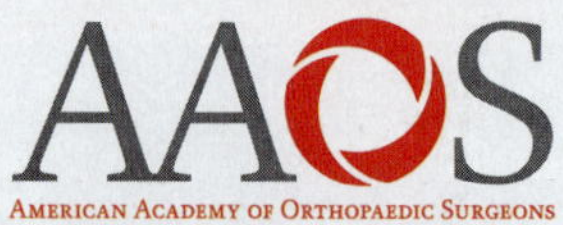

World Headquarters
Jones & Bartlett Learning
25 Mall Road
Burlington, MA 01803
978-443-5000
info@jblearning.com
www.jblearning.com
www.psglearning.com

Editorial Credits
Chief Commercial Officer: Anna Salt Troise, MBA
Director, Publishing: Hans J. Koelsch, PhD
Senior Manager, Editorial: Lisa Claxton Moore

Jones & Bartlett Learning books and products are available through most bookstores and online booksellers. To contact the Jones & Bartlett Learning Public Safety Group directly, call 800-832-0034, fax 978-443-8000, or visit our website, www.psglearning.com.

Substantial discounts on bulk quantities of Jones & Bartlett Learning publications are available to corporations, professional associations, and other qualified organizations. For details and specific discount information, contact the special sales department at Jones & Bartlett Learning via the above contact information or send an email to specialsales@jblearning.com.

32936-0

Production Credits
Vice President, Innovative Learning and Assessment Solutions: Ada Woo
Senior Director, Content Production and Delivery: Christine Emerton
Director, Product: Cathy Esperti
Product Manager, EMS: Jameel Sylvia
Manager, Content Development: Tiffany Sliter
Content Manager: Ashley Procum
Content Coordinator: Samantha Gillespie
Development Editor: Heather Ehlers
Manager, Intellectual Properties and Content Production: Kristen Rogers
Content Production Manager: John Fuller
Senior Intellectual Property Specialist (eBook): Colleen Lamy
Senior Product Marketing Manager: Susanne Walker
Director, Product Fulfillment: Aaron McKinzie
Purchasing Manager: Wendy Kilborn
Composition: S4Carlisle Publishing Services
Cover Design: MPS Limited
Text Design: MPS Limited
Media Developer: Faith Brosnan
Intellectual Property Specialist: Robin Silverman
Cover Image: © wilpunt/E+/Getty Images
Printing and Binding: Lakeside Book Company

Library of Congress Cataloging-in-Publication Data
Library of Congress Cataloging-in-Publication Data unavailable at time of printing.
LCCN: 2026941169

6048

Printed in the United States of America
30 29 28 27 26 10 9 8 7 6 5 4 3 2 1

Brief Contents

Contents

Skill Sheets

Welcome to ECSI

ECSI Overview

Welcome to the Emergency Care and Safety Institute (ECSI)! ECSI is an organization committed to providing the best possible cardiopulmonary resuscitation and first aid training for audiences of all backgrounds. It offers affordable, evidence-based training materials and resources as well as flexible course delivery options to meet the diverse needs of the communities it serves. ECSI's goal is to give educators the tools and support they need—from physical textbooks to eBooks, instructor toolkits, online interactive courses, blended hybrid courses, exceptional customer service, and more—to allow them to focus on what truly matters: training others to save lives.

Audiences

ECSI provides CPR, first aid, and other safety-related training solutions at a variety of levels for a range of audiences. Courses at the professional level lead to certifications that meet job-related requirements as defined by hundreds of regulatory authorities throughout the world. Courses at the general public level are for those interested in learning first aid and CPR for personal reasons. ECSI courses have received regulatory approvals for various categories and are delivered throughout an ever-increasing range of industries and markets worldwide, including (but not limited to) secondary and higher education school systems, community education programs, scouting groups, business and industry, government agencies, public safety agencies, hospitals, and private training companies.

Adherence to Treatment Recommendations

ECSI programs are built on the most recent evidence-based treatment recommendations published by the International Liaison Committee on Resuscitation (ILCOR), known as the Consensus on Science with Treatment Recommendations (CoSTR). They also meet the American Heart Association (AHA) Emergency Cardiovascular Care (ECC) Guidelines and—where applicable—the Stop the Bleed campaign. Consistency with these guidelines ensures the most current and effective lifesaving techniques are being taught in all ECSI programs.

Inclusion of Graphic Imagery

All ECSI training programs contain graphic images and descriptions, including but not limited to bloody wounds, burns, traumatic injuries, and amputations. Some images use moulage, including simulated injuries and artificial blood, while others are real and depict actual injuries. Both types of imagery are intentionally included to reflect the realities of medical emergencies while supporting skill development and emotional preparedness in a safe learning environment.

Exposure to realistic imagery during training is an important part of first aid and CPR education. It can help learners recognize serious injuries, maintain focus under stress, and develop the confidence needed to respond effectively in real-world situations where injuries may be visually distressing. Familiarity with these conditions during training supports better decision making and emotional readiness when providing care to injured individuals.

We recognize that graphic content may be distressing for some individuals. Emotional reactions to this material are normal and valid. Learners are encouraged to engage with the content in a way that feels manageable, take breaks as needed, and use available resources to support both their education and personal well-being.

Partner Organizations

ECSI programs are offered in partnership with the American Academy of Orthopaedic Surgeons (AAOS) and the American College of Emergency Physicians (ACEP), two of the most renowned medical organizations in the world.

AAOS, the world's largest medical association of musculoskeletal specialists, is known as the original name in emergency medical services (EMS) publishing, putting out the first EMS textbook in 1971. ACEP is widely recognized as the leading name in all of emergency medicine.

These organizations provide medical direction to ECSI and stand behind ECSI's training materials. For more, visit www.aaos.org and www.acep.org.

For More Information

Want to learn more about ECSI, catch up on the lifesaving training blog, take a course, or become an ECSI Instructor? Visit www.ecsinstitute.org today!

Acknowledgments

The authors, the series editor, the Jones & Bartlett Learning Public Safety Group, the American Academy of Orthopaedic Surgeons, and the American College of Emergency Physicians would like to thank all of the reviewers and contributors who generously offered their time, expertise, and talent to the making of this ninth edition.

Reviewers

Ninth Edition Reviewers

Julia Aguiar, BSN, RN
Manlius Pebble Hill
Syracuse, New York

Matt Crouse
Nixa Parks and Recreation
Nixa, Missouri

Andrew Desmond
Training Center Instructor
AGDESMOND, LLC
Newark, New Jersey

Kathy Devlin
Owner
Dev-Tac, LLC
New Jersey

Raffaele M. Di Giorgio
Co-Founder, CEO
Global Options & Solutions

Victor Flanagan, AEMT
Training Center Coordinator
Great Falls Council BSA
Buffalo, New York

Denise Gerhart, HHP
FEMA Preparedness Instructor
ECSI Life Support Instructor
Sapere Aude
Hutchinson, Kansas

Linda J. Gosselin, MS, REMT IC, Ed
MECTA Academy
Millbury, Massachusetts

Gregory Harter, MD, FAAFP
Winnebago Boy Scouts
Waterloo, Iowa

Frank Kachurak, MS IT
Clinical Coordinator
Centre County Public Safety Training Center
Pleasant Gap, Pennsylvania
Managing Partner
Halligan Training, LLC
Rebersburg, Pennsylvania

Kevin Leffler
Wilderness First Aid Instructor
First Aid Instructor
CPR and AED Instructor
Appalachian Outfitters
Peninsula, Ohio

Barb Libstorff, BS
Health and Safety Consultant
Safety Plus LLC
Monclova, Ohio

Mark McCoy
Learning and Performance Center
Chesterfield County, Virginia

Joseph McCue, LMT
New Hampshire Department of Transportation
Concord, New Hampshire

Vincent Montefusco
SMART Medical Training
Spring Hill, Florida

Tresa Radermacher
SFA, CPR, AED Instructor
Dyer, Indiana

Amy S. Riggio, MEd
Loudoun County Public Schools
Ashburn, Virginia

Mark Schaefer
Owner/Instructor
Simple CPR, LLC
Colorado Springs, Colorado

Wayne Stephens, NREMT, FAWM
Mid-Minnesota EMS Education
Brandon, Minnesota

Bob Surrusco, LTC GaSDF
Executive Director, Owner
The Readiness Professionals

Joseph Varacalle, Jr
Boy Scout Troop 26
Baltimore, Maryland

Eighth Edition Reviewers

Ken Bartz, AEMT
EMS Instructor Coordinator
Southwest Wisconsin Technical College
Fennimore, Wisconsin

Kent Courtney
Paramedic, Firefighter, Rescue Technician, Educator
Essential Safety Training and Consulting
Lake Montezuma, Arizona

Chance Cummings
Lieutenant, Paramedic, EMS Liaison Officer
Starkville Fire Department
Starkville, Mississippi

James W. Fogal, MA, NRP
Auburn University
Auburn, Alabama

Fidel O. Garcia
Paramedic
Professional EMS Education
Grand Junction, Colorado

Michele M. Hoffman, MS, Ed, RN, NREMT
James City County Fire Department
Williamsburg, Virginia

Benjamin McKenna, MA
AHA CTC Coordinator
University of South Alabama
Mobile, Alabama

Gregory S. Neiman, MS, NRP, NCEE
EMS Liaison
Virginia Commonwealth University Health
Richmond, Virginia

William H. Turner, MS, NRP, EMSI
Assistant Professor, Director of Emergency Medical Technology
Shawnee State University
Portsmouth, Ohio

Josh Weiner, NRP, FP-C
Minneapolis, Minnesota

Raymond C. Whatley, Jr, MBA, NRP, CEM
Emergency Health Services Program
George Washington University
Washington, District of Columbia

Christopher C. Williams, PhD, NRP
Guilford County EMS
Greensboro, North Carolina

Photo and Video Services

The team wishes to thank all the **models** who brought the videos to life, including **Rich Nydam**, education coordinator at Worcester EMS, who shared his subject matter expertise, professional direction, and training facility during our photography and videography projects. It is a privilege to collaborate with a valued member of our community!

Additionally, the team extends their gratitude to **Curt Fetter**, director, producer, editor, and owner of Dvee Media Productions for his professional direction and expertise in capturing both photography and videography for this and many other Public Safety Group projects.

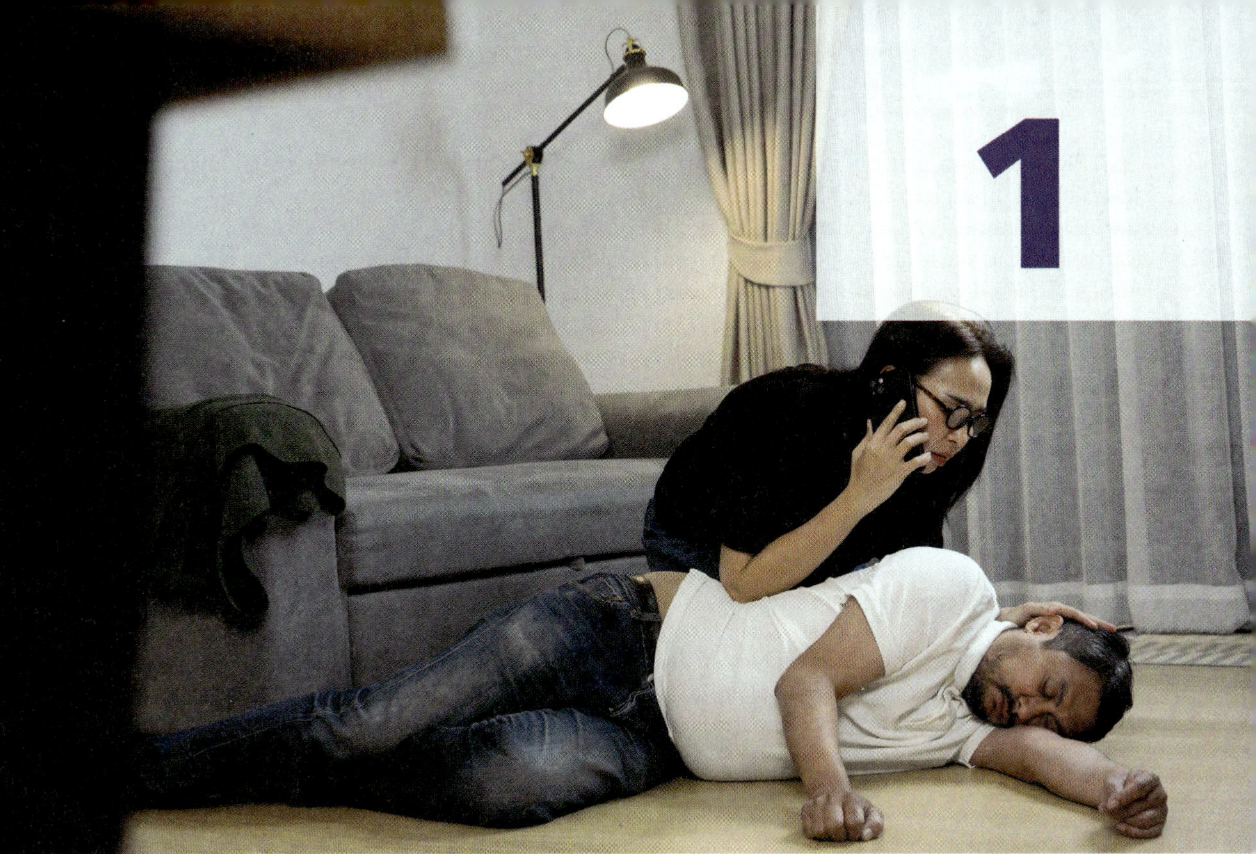

© jittawit.21/iStock/Getty Images Plus/Getty Images

Preparing to Help

Introduction

Heart disease is the number one cause of death in the United States (and many other countries). More than 350,000 cardiac arrests occur outside of a hospital each year, but fewer than 10% of people survive. High-quality cardiopulmonary resuscitation (CPR), started immediately after the arrest, can double or triple the chance of survival. However, only about 40% of people who experience sudden cardiac arrest receive immediate help from bystanders before emergency medical services (EMS) arrives. The aim of this manual is to increase the number of people who feel comfortable providing CPR to a person in need, which in turn will increase the percentage of people receiving CPR and thus the survival rate.

CHAPTER AT A GLANCE

CPR, on its own, generally will not restart a heart that has stopped beating. Instead, it manually circulates blood through the body so that oxygen continues to be delivered to vital organs and keeps them alive until defibrillation and definitive care can be provided. Defibrillation involves administering an electric shock to the heart to correct an abnormal rhythm (heartbeat). An automated external defibrillator (AED) is a device that can analyze a person's heart rhythm and provide a shock, if necessary. AEDs are designed to be user friendly and can be operated by people with minimal training. This manual will outlines the basic operational principles that all AED models use.

Choking is the fourth most common cause of unintentional injury death, with more than 5,000 people dying each year. The highest rates are in those younger than 5 years and those older than 70 years. On average, more than 15,000 children younger than 14 years are treated in emergency departments annually for choking-related incidents. This manual discusses care for airway obstruction for adults, children, and infants, which includes alternating back blows and abdominal/chest thrusts.

Deciding to Help

At one time or another, everyone will have to decide whether or not to help someone. Unless the decision to act in an emergency is considered well in advance of an actual emergency, the many obstacles that make it difficult or unpleasant for you to help are almost certain to impede action. One important strategy that many people use to avoid action is to refuse (consciously or unconsciously) to acknowledge the emergency. Many emergencies do not look obvious, like those portrayed on television, and the uncertainty surrounding an actual emergency can make it easier for people to avoid acknowledging the situation as an emergency. Another consideration is something called the "bystander effect," which is a psychological theory that states that people are less likely to offer help if other people are around. Although there are many variables that affect the likelihood of a person intervening, the basic idea is that when an individual is in a group, they are less likely to help in an emergency because of the assumption that someone else will help.

One of the biggest struggles people experience with regard to helping is lack of confidence in their abilities. Despite their training, concern that something may go wrong or they may do the wrong thing is a major barrier when it comes to approaching and helping a person who needs care. So long as you recognize the limits of your knowledge and abilities, and stay within them, your actions will be more likely to help than harm. If you are ever faced with an emergency that requires care you cannot provide, or you do not know what to do, immediately call 9-1-1. Trained emergency dispatchers can provide instructions and help guide you as you provide care.

People are more likely to promptly get involved at the time of an emergency if they have previously considered the possibility of helping others (**FIGURE 1-1**). Thus, the most important time to make the decision to help is before ever encountering an emergency. Deciding to help is an attitude about emergencies and about one's ability to handle them. It is an attitude that takes time to develop and is affected by several factors. To develop this type of proactive attitude, an individual must do the following:

- Understand the importance of helping an injured or suddenly ill person.
- Feel confident about helping someone who is seriously injured or suddenly ill, even if someone else is present.
- Be willing to take the time to help.
- Be able to put the potential risks of helping into perspective.
- Feel comfortable about taking charge, if needed, at an emergency scene. This is accomplished with ongoing competency in your skills training as well as experience, either actual or simulated.
- Feel comfortable about seeing a person who is bleeding or vomiting or who appears unresponsive or dead.

Checking the Scene

Before you approach the person, evaluate the situation. This is often called the scene size-up. It is important to gather as much information as you can to ensure your own safety and the safety of the person you are trying help. Never rush in to help without first confirming that the scene is safe to enter. A scene size-up can be performed in about 10 seconds and involves asking yourself the questions in **FLOWCHART 1-1**.

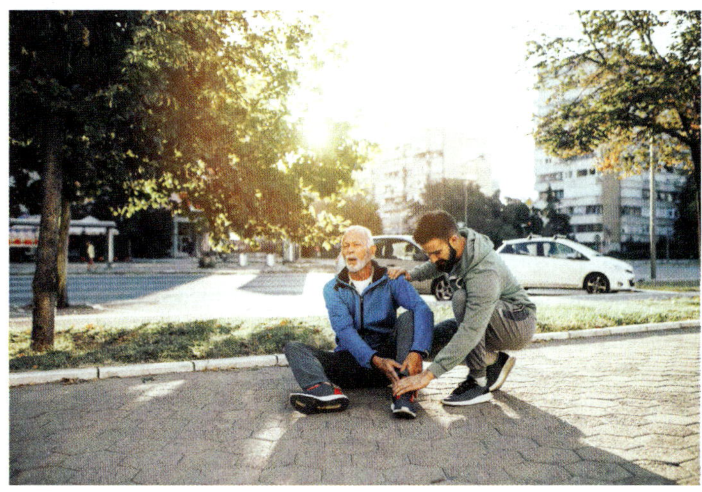

FIGURE 1-1 Be willing to take the time to help.

Flowchart 1-1 Check the Scene

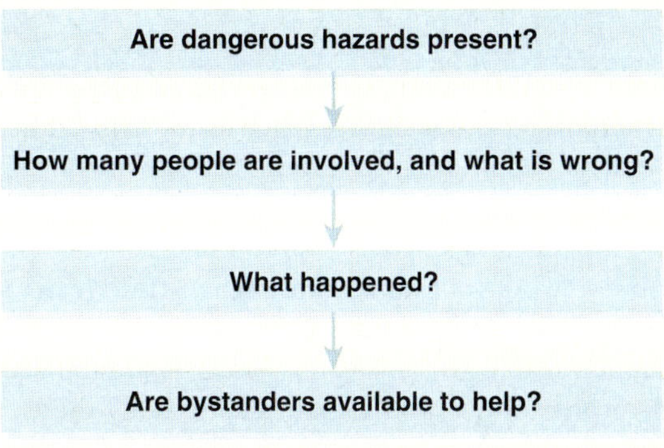

Contacting Emergency Medical Services

If the scene is dangerous or you cannot access the person, call 9-1-1 immediately. Otherwise, you must be able to tell the difference between a minor injury or illness and a life-threatening one. Some signs of serious injury or illness are obvious, even from a distance. These include a motionless person, life-threatening bleeding, or a mechanism of injury that indicates the potential for severe injuries (eg, a vehicle crash with significant damage). If unsure, call 9-1-1 and the trained dispatcher will advise you. It is better to be safe and call 9-1-1 when in doubt.

When you call 9-1-1 (or the local emergency number), the emergency dispatcher will guide you, but the following information is commonly required:

- Your name and the phone number you are calling from. This allows the dispatcher to call you back if you get disconnected.
- The location of the emergency. Be as specific as possible. Give the address, if known, and any intersecting roads, landmarks, or specific location information (eg, "13 Elm Street, in the backyard").
- A description of what happened. State the nature of the emergency, the number of people needing help, and any special conditions.
- A description of the person's condition. Provide a quick description of the signs/symptoms the person is experiencing, plus any care that has been provided.

DO NOT hang up the phone unless the dispatcher instructs you to. Emergency medical dispatchers are trained to provide guidance on initial actions; if possible, put the phone on speaker to free your hands to provide care and follow instructions. If another person was sent to call 9-1-1, have them report back to you so that you know the call was made and you receive any instructions from the dispatcher.

Taking Standard Precautions

Body fluids (such as blood, saliva, and stool) can sometimes carry organisms that are capable of producing illness in an exposed person, such as the following:

- HIV/AIDS
- Hepatitis B virus
- Hepatitis C virus
- Tuberculosis
- Meningitis
- COVID-19

The Centers for Disease Control and Prevention (CDC) developed a set of *standard precautions* designed to help prevent the transmission of infectious diseases such as those listed here. These standard precautions advise you to assume that all people are infected and can spread an organism that poses a risk for transmission of infectious diseases. These protective measures are designed to prevent rescuers from coming into direct contact with infectious agents. Appropriate personal protective equipment (PPE) should always be worn. Be sure to wash your hands thoroughly after every contact with an ill or injured person, even if you wore gloves. Also wash or rinse any exposed areas, including your eyes, nose, and mouth. If soap and water are unavailable, use an alcohol-based hand sanitizer—but only on your hands.

If, despite taking standard precautions, you are exposed to body fluids, contact your primary care physician for follow-up. If you are at work, inform your supervisor so that postexposure protocols can be initiated (if necessary). Early treatment can prevent the development of certain infections.

Personal Protective Equipment

Avoid contact with blood and other body fluids by putting on PPE, which includes:

- Disposable medical exam gloves (use latex-free gloves, if possible; nitrile gloves are recommended; **FIGURE 1-2**)
- Eye protection (goggles or face shield)
- Mouth-to-barrier device when giving CPR (**FIGURE 1-3**)
- Face covering (face mask or face shield) to prevent disease transmission (**FIGURE 1-4**)

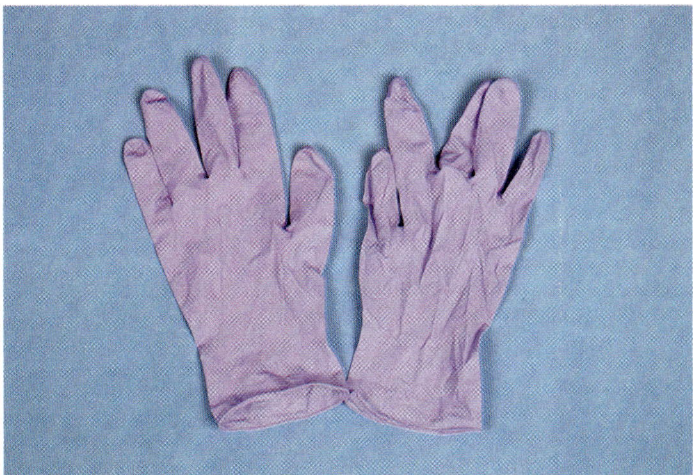

FIGURE 1-2 Disposable gloves.

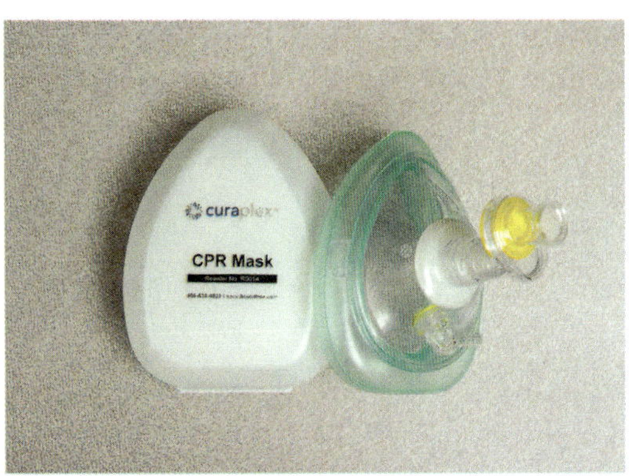

A

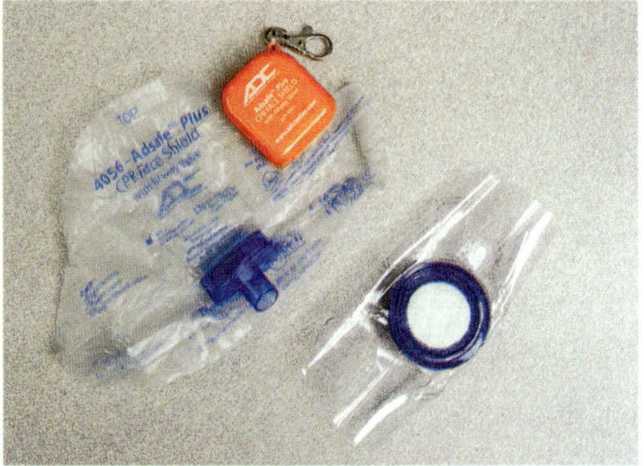

B

FIGURE 1-3 Mouth-to-barrier devices. **A.** Mask. **B.** Face shields.

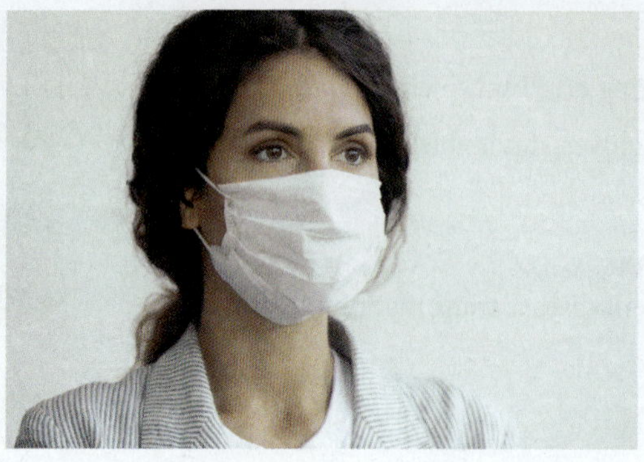

A

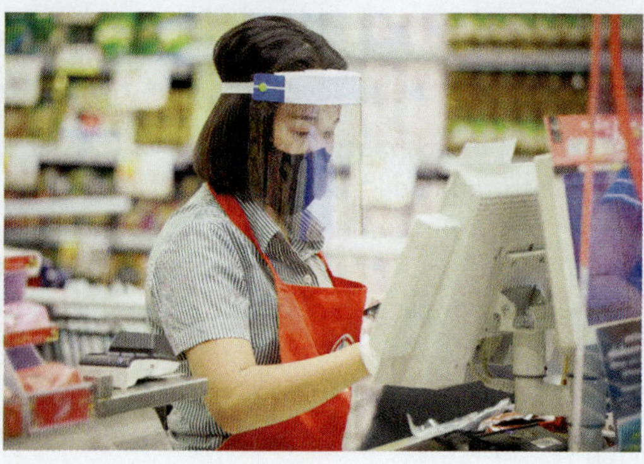

B

FIGURE 1-4 **A.** Face mask for public health. **B.** Face shield for public health.
A: © fizkes/Shutterstock; **B:** © pixfly/Shutterstock

Washing Your Hands

Handwashing is one of the simplest, yet most effective, ways to control disease transmission. Wash your hands as follows after giving first aid (even if gloves were worn; **FIGURE 1-5**):

1. Wet your hands with clean, running water (warm or cool) and apply soap.
2. Lather by rubbing hands together. Be sure to get the backs of your hands, between all fingers, and under your nails.
3. Scrub all hand surfaces for at least 20 seconds.
4. Rinse off the soap completely with clean, running water.
5. With the water still running, dry your hands with a clean towel or paper towel. Avoid touching the water faucet by using a towel to turn off the water.

A hand sanitizer containing at least 60% alcohol can be used if soap and water are not immediately available (**FIGURE 1-6**), but you should still properly wash your hands with soap and water as soon as possible.

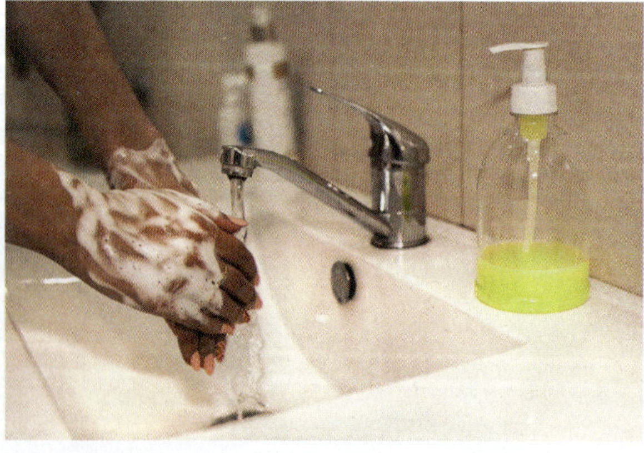

FIGURE 1-5 Handwashing.
© diy13/Shutterstock

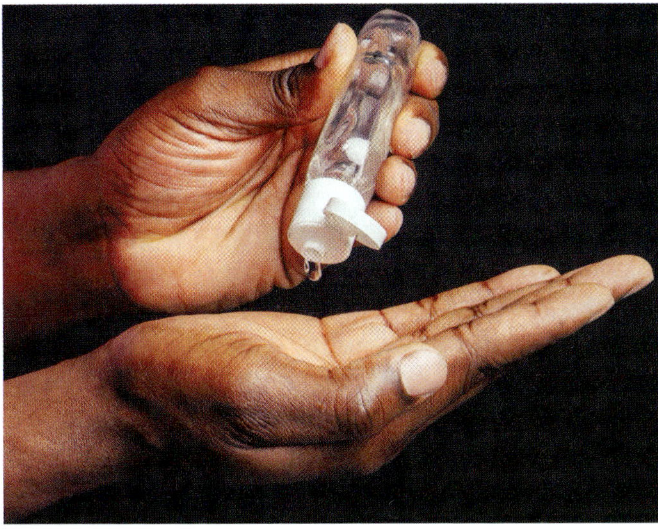

FIGURE 1-6 Hand sanitizer.

Legal Considerations

Most people believe helping others is the right thing to do. However, you are not legally required to help another person unless you have a legal duty to act (**FIGURE 1-7**) such as in the following situations:

- Employment requires it (eg, job description)
- Preexisting relationship exists (eg, parent–child, teacher–student, driver–passenger)

Good Samaritan Laws

Good Samaritan laws apply to anyone who provides voluntary, unpaid care in an emergency situation, such as first aid and CPR providers. They do not apply to those with a legal duty to act, such as emergency medical technicians or firefighters. Good Samaritan laws provide reasonable protection against lawsuits and encourage people to help others during an emergency. Laws are different from state to state, but, in general, the following conditions must be met:

- You are acting with good intentions.
- You are providing care without expectation of compensation.
- You are acting within the scope of your training.
- You are not acting in a grossly negligent (reckless) manner.

Negligent actions include the following:

- Giving substandard care
- Withholding care when you have a legal duty to act
- Intentionally causing injury or harm
- Exceeding your level of training
- Abandoning the person (starting care and then stopping or leaving without ensuring that a rescuer with the same or a higher level of training will continue to care for the person)

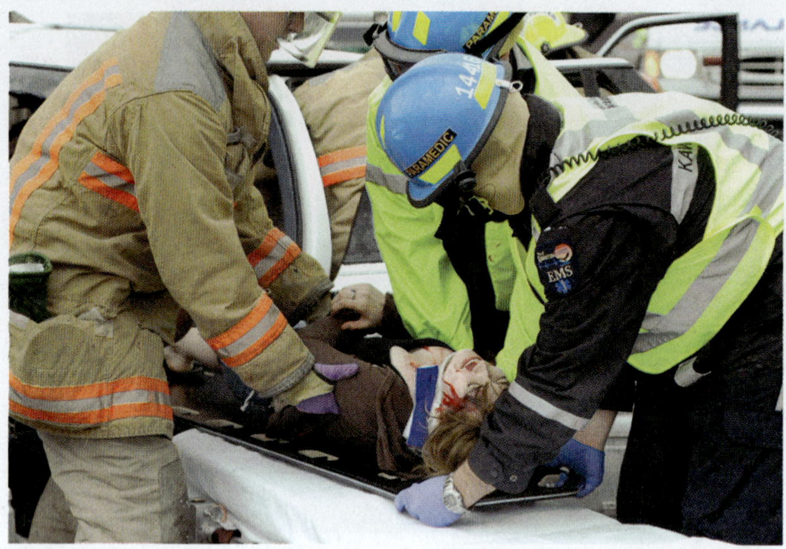

FIGURE 1-7 Firefighters and paramedics are examples of providers who have a legal duty to act.

Confidential Information

In the course of providing care, you might learn confidential information. It is important to be extremely cautious about revealing information that you may learn while caring for someone. The law recognizes that people have the right to privacy. Do not discuss what you know with anyone other than those who have a medical need to know.

Consent

You must obtain the person's consent (permission) before providing care. Touching another person without their consent is illegal and could be grounds for a lawsuit. If the person is an adult and responsive (eg, choking but conscious), ask if you can help. For an unresponsive person (eg, not breathing and in need of CPR), you can assume that they would consent to care if they were able to; this is known as *implied consent*. Do not withhold lifesaving care in this situation.

Except for certain instances, children cannot legally provide consent. However, if the child is unresponsive or is experiencing a life-threatening emergency (eg, severe airway obstruction), you can assume implied consent and provide care.

Emotional Considerations

An emergency involving a cardiac arrest or airway obstruction can be an incredibly stressful experience. Both are time-sensitive conditions and require an immediate response. Bystanders may be panicking and demanding you act quickly. This is where your training is helpful: Knowing what to do and how to respond can help you stay focused and calm.

Resilience

You can also work to improve your personal resilience. *Resilience* is the ability to cope with stress without experiencing lasting harm. While some people are naturally more resilient than others, it is a skill that can be learned. Factors that can improve resilience include the following:

- Maintaining a positive outlook
- Maintaining social connections
- Developing healthy coping mechanisms
- Seeking professional support when needed

Postcare Reactions

After providing CPR, a person might feel an emotional letdown. This situation is frequently overlooked. A stressful event can be psychologically overwhelming and can result in a condition known as posttraumatic stress disorder (PTSD). Its symptoms include depression and flashbacks of the event.

Discussing your feelings, fears, and reactions (while maintaining the privacy of the person[s] you helped) within 24 to 72 hours of helping at a cardiac arrest or airway obstruction emergency helps prevent later emotional conditions. You could discuss your feelings with a trusted friend, a mental health professional, or a religious or spiritual mentor. Bringing out your feelings quickly can relieve personal anxieties and stress.

You must also accept that, unfortunately, you cannot treat or save everyone. Some situations may have outcomes that are simply beyond anyone's control, no matter how prepared or well-intentioned they are. However, CPR training puts you in a much better position to confidently and effectively respond. The information in this course will give you the tools you need to stay calm, confidently take action, and possibly make a life-changing difference. Even when the outcome is not what you may have hoped for, your effort matters. Being prepared can make all the difference.

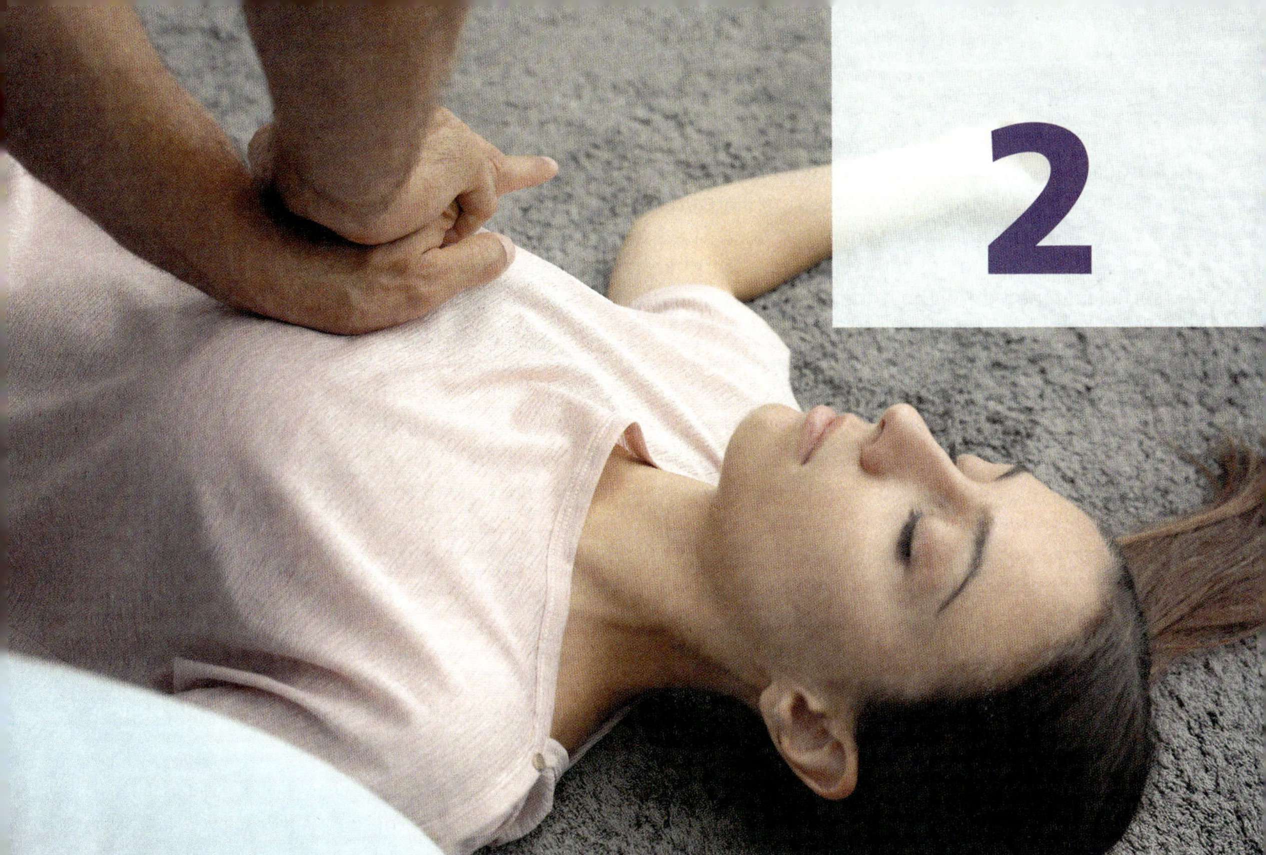

© New Africa/Shutterstock

Cardiopulmonary Resuscitation

CHAPTER AT A GLANCE

- Heart Attack Versus Cardiac Arrest
- Cardiopulmonary Resuscitation

Heart Attack Versus Cardiac Arrest

The terms *heart attack* and *cardiac arrest* confuse many people because they are, in fact, different conditions. To provide the best care, you must be able to tell them apart.

A heart attack happens when the blood supply to the heart muscle is suddenly reduced or blocked. In most cases, the heart continues to beat and the person remains responsive. They will often (though not always) report chest pain or discomfort, among other symptoms. Left untreated, a heart attack can lead to cardiac arrest. This is why a person experiencing a heart attack needs immediate professional medical care.

A cardiac arrest occurs when the heart stops pumping blood. This happens because the heart stops beating or beats too quickly (ventricular tachycardia) or irregularly (ventricular fibrillation) to circulate sufficient blood throughout the body. It is one of the leading causes of death. A person experiencing cardiac arrest will be unresponsive and may stop breathing (or only gasp for air).

Definitive treatment for cardiac arrest is to either restart the heart or correct the irregular heart rate. Cardiopulmonary resuscitation (CPR) is the set of lifesaving skills necessary to help a person in cardiac arrest until emergency medical services (EMS) arrive to take over. Basically, CPR manually circulates blood through the body to keep blood flowing to the body's organs. This helps provide oxygen to vital organs such as the brain and heart to keep them alive. Receiving immediate CPR after a cardiac arrest can triple a person's chances of survival.

One reason why bystanders do not perform CPR is that they worry about hurting the person (eg, breaking ribs). While this can happen, any harm done is less severe than having a nonfunctioning heart, which is always fatal.

An automated external defibrillator (AED) is an electronic device that analyzes the heart rhythm and if necessary prompts the rescuer to deliver an electric shock, known as defibrillation, to the heart of a person in cardiac arrest. This electrical shock is designed to reestablish an effective rhythm and thus improve blood flow.

Cardiopulmonary Resuscitation

For a life-threatening condition such as cardiac arrest, doing something is always better than doing nothing! This is not only the case for the person requiring care, but also for your benefit as the CPR provider. Even if unsuccessful, you will know that you tried everything you could to save the person's life.

Adult or Child CPR

When you see a motionless adult or child, scan the scene for hazards that could endanger your life. Being injured yourself could prevent you from providing CPR. In other words, take standard precautions (see pp. 5–6).

If there is life-threatening bleeding, quickly control it (or have someone else to control it) using either direct pressure or a manufactured tourniquet (see Appendix B).

Use the **RAB-CAB** mnemonic to remember the sequence of what to do when providing adult or child CPR. RAB-CAB stands for:

R = Responsive?
A = Activate EMS and get an AED
B = Breathing?
C = Compressions
A = Airway open
B = Breaths

R = Responsive?

Tap the person's shoulder and shout, "Are you okay?" to determine if the person is responsive or unresponsive. If the person is unresponsive (eg, does not answer, move, or moan), continue to the next step, *A = Activate EMS and get an AED.*

A = Activate EMS and Get an AED

Shout for nearby help.

If...	Then...
Someone comes to help.	▪ Have them activate EMS by calling 9-1-1 or the local emergency number and get an AED, if readily available, while you continue providing care. If the person is using a mobile phone, turn on speakerphone to hear the dispatcher.
You are alone and the person is an adult.	▪ If you have a phone, call 9-1-1 and get an AED, if readily available. Turn on speakerphone to hear the dispatcher and leave your hands free to provide care. ▪ If you do not have a phone, leave the person to call 9-1-1 and get an AED, if readily available. After making the call, return and continue providing care.
You are alone and the person is a child (between age 1 and puberty).	▪ If you have a phone, call 9-1-1 and follow the dispatcher's instructions. Turn on speakerphone to hear the dispatcher and leave your hands free to provide care. ▪ If you do not have a phone, give 5 sets of CPR (30 compressions and 2 rescue breaths per set) before leaving to call 9-1-1 and before getting an AED, if readily available.

B = Breathing?

Observe the person from neck to waist for movement (rise and fall); take 5 to 10 seconds. **DO NOT** check for a pulse. Doing so is often unreliable and only delays lifesaving care.

If the person is not breathing or is only gasping (may sound like a quick inhalation or like a groan or snore), place them faceup on a flat, firm surface and continue to the next step, *C = Compressions.*

C = Compressions

Give chest compressions.

When possible, place the person on a flat, firm surface on their back. Then, perform compressions with the person's chest at about the level of your knees (eg, person on floor, ground).

1. Move enough clothing to locate the correct hand position for compressions and to apply an AED when it arrives on the scene. Hand placement varies slightly depending on the age and size of the person:
    a. For adults and children, place the heel of one hand on the center of the person's chest and on the lower half of their breastbone (sternum).
    b. For an adult, place your other hand on top of the first one with your fingers interlocked. Hold your fingers off the person's chest and point them directly away from you (**FIGURE 2-1**). **DO NOT** cross your hands.
    c. For a child, use just one hand (**FIGURE 2-2**). However, if the child is large or you are small, use two hands as for adults.

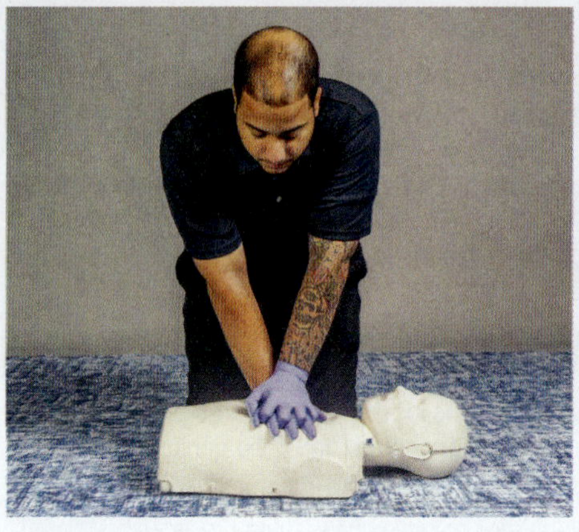

A

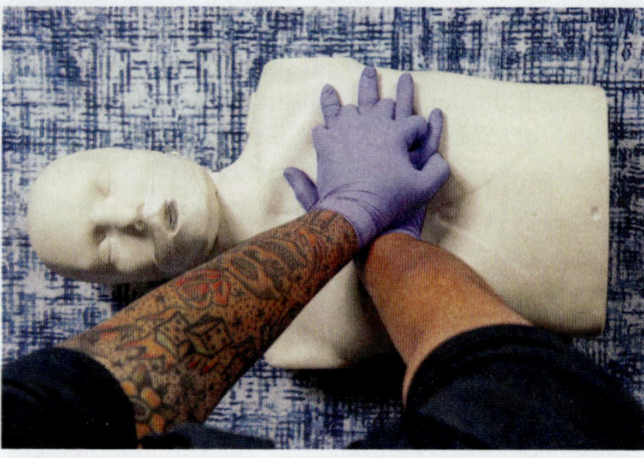

B

FIGURE 2-1 For adult CPR, place the heel of one hand on the center of the chest, on the lower half of the breastbone. Place your other hand on top, interlock your fingers, and keep them lifted up off the chest. **A.** Frontal view. **B.** Overhead view (CPR provider's point of view).

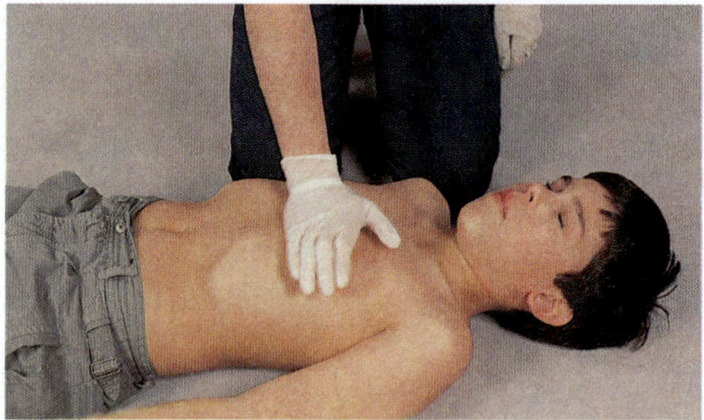

FIGURE 2-2 For child CPR, place the heel of one hand on the center of the chest, in between the nipples.

2. Keep your arm(s) straight and elbow(s) locked, with your shoulders positioned directly over your hand(s).
3. Push straight down on the breastbone (sternum).
   a. Push hard: Use your upper body weight, not just your arms, to compress the chest, pushing at least 2 inches (5 cm) for an adult and about 2 inches or one-third the depth of the chest for a child.
   b. Push fast: Give 30 compressions at a rate of 100 to 120 compressions per minute. To maintain the compression rate, follow the beat of the Bee Gees song "Stayin' Alive," the beat from a CPR smartphone app that was previously installed and is quickly accessible, or a dispatcher's directions heard over a mobile phone speaker.
   c. Push smoothly: **DO NOT** bounce or jab. **DO NOT** stop at the top or bottom of a compression. **DO NOT** rock back and forth.
4. Allow the chest to fully recoil after each compression. **DO NOT** lean on the chest.

A = Airway Open

Open the person's airway using the head tilt–chin lift maneuver (**FIGURE 2-3**):

1. Take your hand nearest the person's head and place it on their forehead; apply pressure to tilt the head back.
2. Place two fingers of your other hand under the bony part of the person's jaw (near the chin) and lift. Avoid pressing on the soft tissues under the jaw.
3. Tilt the head backward.

In cases of suspected spinal injury, **DO NOT** move the person's head or neck. *Carefully* use the jaw-thrust maneuver (**FIGURE 2-4**) instead:

1. With both hands, one on each side, place your index and middle fingers behind the angles of the jaw and your thumbs on the cheekbones.
2. Move the lower jaw forward without tilting the head back.
3. If the jaw-thrust maneuver is unsuccessful, *carefully* perform the head tilt–chin lift maneuver. The person will die without an open airway.

DO NOT apply a cervical collar or other immobilization device on people with suspected spinal injuries. Instead, manually stabilize the head and neck in the position they were found until EMS personnel take over.

B = Breaths

Give two rescue breaths while keeping the person's airway open:

1. When possible, use a mouth-to-barrier device to prevent potential disease transmission. If not using a barrier device, pinch the person's nose shut and make a tight seal with your mouth on the person's mouth. If using a barrier device, make a tight seal on the mouth-to-barrier device. If unwilling or unable to give rescue breaths (ie, seriously injured mouth, ineffective seal, mouth cannot be opened), give compression-only CPR.
2. Give two rescue breaths while keeping the airway open, each lasting 1 second and just strong enough to raise the chest. **DO NOT** blow too forcefully or for too long. Allow for chest deflation after each rescue breath. Take a normal breath for yourself after each rescue breath.

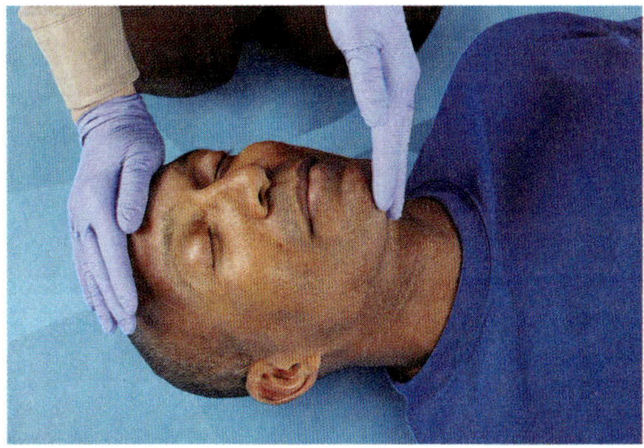

FIGURE 2-3 Open the person's airway with the head tilt–chin lift maneuver if a spinal injury is not suspected.

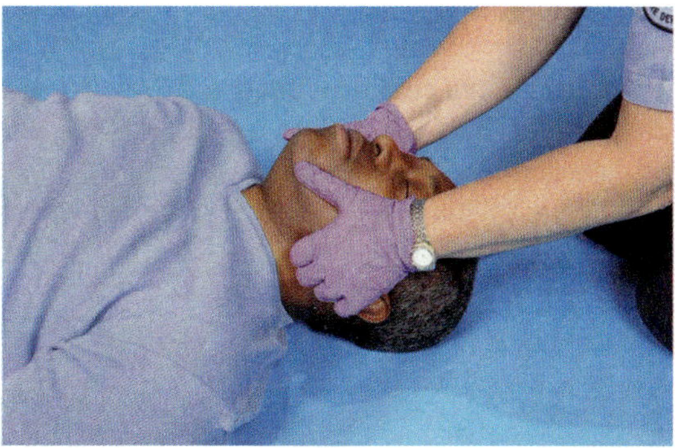

FIGURE 2-4 Use the jaw-thrust maneuver to open the person's airway without extending the neck when a spinal injury is suspected.

3. Watch for chest rise to determine if your rescue breaths go in.

If...	Then...
You see the chest rise after giving two rescue breaths.	Give sets of 30 chest compressions followed by 2 rescue breaths.
The first rescue breath does not cause the chest to rise.	Retilt the person's head and give a second rescue breath.
You retilt the head and the second rescue breath still does not allow the chest to rise.	▪ An object may be blocking the person's airway. Follow steps for an unresponsive person with an airway obstruction (p. 34).
You cannot use the person's mouth (eg, seriously injured mouth, ineffective seal, mouth cannot be opened).	▪ Open the person's airway as previously described. ▪ Seal your mouth around the person's nose and breathe out. ▪ Alternatively, use compression-only CPR (discussed later).
The person vomits or there is fluid in the mouth.	▪ Roll the person onto their side and clear the mouth using a gloved finger or piece of gauze. Be sure to keep the body aligned (nose and navel always pointing in the same direction) to avoid worsening a possible spinal injury (this usually requires more than one person). ▪ Roll the person onto their back and continue care.

4. Continue sets of 30 chest compressions and 2 rescue breaths until:
   - An AED arrives (follow the manufacturer's directions for pad placement). After the AED pads are placed on the exposed chest, the AED will advise when and if to shock and if CPR should be continued.
   - The person begins breathing.
   - Another rescuer (eg, EMS personnel, trained first aid or CPR provider) replaces you and gives CPR.
   - The scene becomes unsafe. If possible, the person should be quickly moved to a nearby safer location before continuing CPR.
   - You are alone and become physically exhausted and are unable to continue.

If another person is present, they could help by giving chest compressions while you give rescue breaths, or vice versa. If the other person is not trained in CPR, you can coach them on how to perform chest compressions and how to give rescue breaths. Switching places after every 5 sets (about every 2 minutes) helps avoid fatigue.

The concern about contracting a disease from giving rescue breaths can be remedied by (1) giving compression-only CPR or (2) having both rescuers use their own mouth-to-barrier device while giving rescue breaths.

Refer to **SKILL SHEET 2-1** for the steps and techniques for adult or child CPR.

Skill Sheet 2-1 Adult and Child CPR

Note: Whenever possible, use a mouth-to-barrier device to prevent disease transmission. Always take standard precautions.

Use the **RAB-CAB** mnemonic to remember what to do.

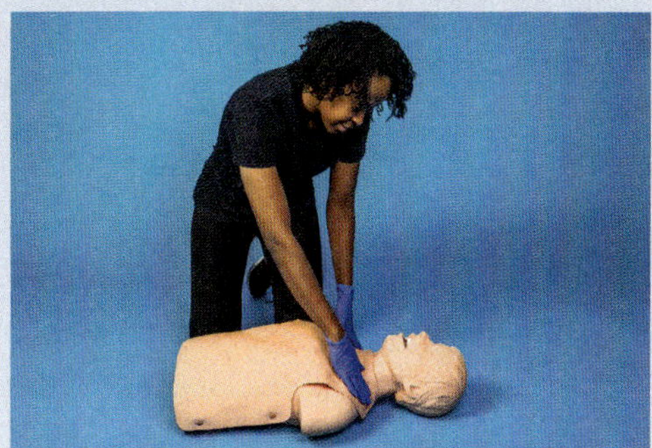

1 **R = Responsive?**

Tap the person's shoulder and shout, "Are you okay?"

a. If the person does not respond, continue to the next step, *A = Activate EMS and get and AED.*

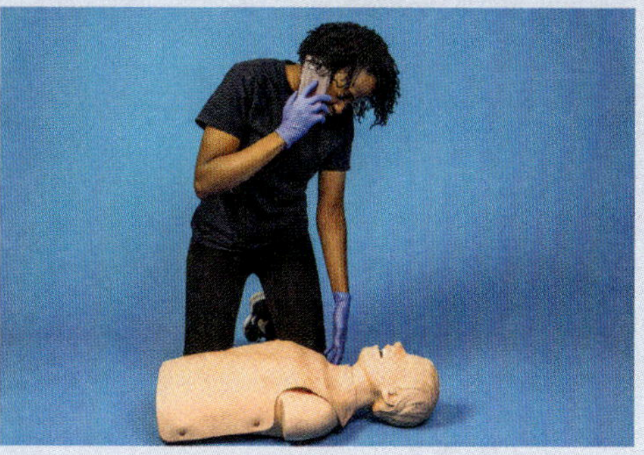

2 **A = Activate EMS and get an AED.**

a. Shout for nearby help.
b. If someone responds, have them call 9-1-1 and get an AED while you provide care.
c. If no one comes and you are alone with an adult, call 9-1-1 and put the phone on speaker mode so that you can prepare to follow the dispatcher's instructions. If a phone is not available, leave the person to locate a phone and get an AED, if available and quickly obtained.
d. If no one comes and you are alone with a child, give 5 sets of 30 chest compressions and 2 rescue breaths before calling 9-1-1. Respiratory arrest is a more common cause of cardiac arrest in children, and immediate CPR is crucial.

(*continues*)

Skill Sheet 2-1 Adult and Child CPR *(continued)*

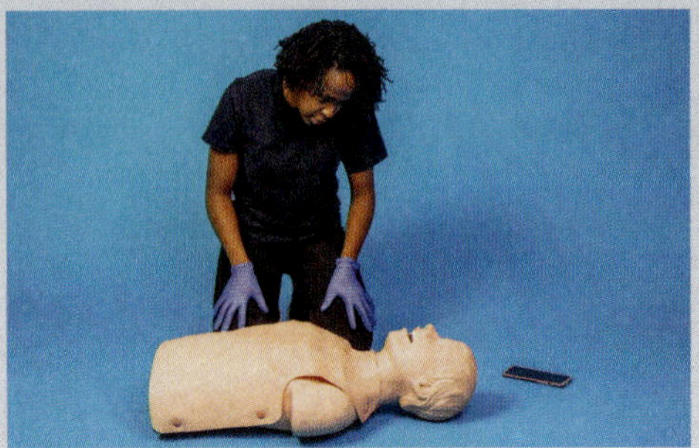

3 **B = Breathing?**

CPR providers should not check for a pulse.

a. Place the person faceup on a flat, firm surface.
b. Take 5 to 10 seconds to observe the person from neck to waist for movement (rise and fall).
c. If the person is not breathing or is only gasping, continue to the next step, *C = Compressions*.

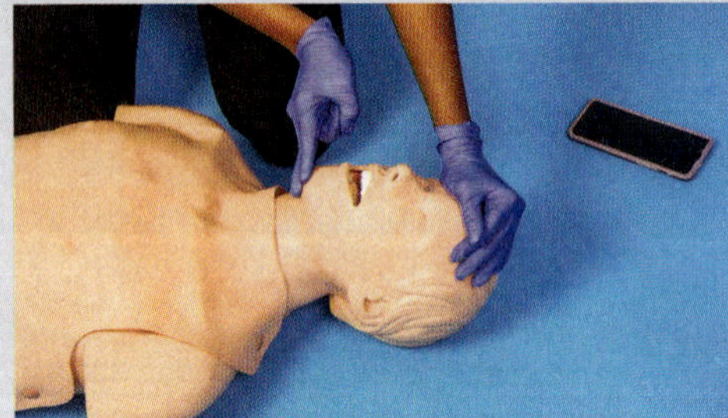

5 **A = Airway open.**

Open the person's airway with the head tilt–chin lift maneuver:

a. Take your hand nearest to the person's head and place it on their forehead; apply pressure to tilt the head back.
b. Place two fingers of your other hand under the bony part of the person's jaw (near the chin) and lift. Avoid pressing on soft tissues under the jaw.
c. Tilt the head backward.

If a spinal injury is suspected, perform the jaw-thrust maneuver (see Figure 2-4). If unsuccessful, carefully perform the head tilt–chin lift maneuver. The person will die without an open airway.

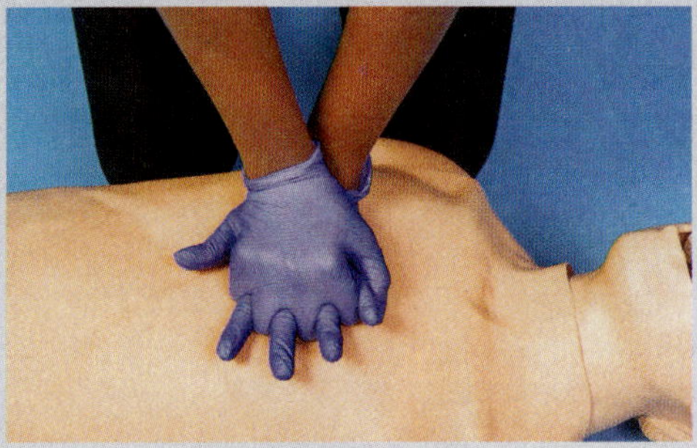

4 **C = Compressions.**

Provide chest compressions:

a. Move enough clothing to locate the correct hand position for compressions and where to apply the AED pads when it arrives on the scene.
b. For an adult:
   - Place the heel of one hand on the center of the person's chest and on the lower half of their breastbone (sternum).
   - Place your other hand on top of the first one with your fingers interlocked. Hold your fingers off the person's chest and point them directly away from you.
c. For a child:
   - Use one hand only; however, depending on the child's size and your size, using two hands may be necessary.
d. Keep your arms straight and elbows locked, with your shoulders positioned directly over your hands.
e. Push hard and straight down on the breastbone (sternum), at least 2 inches (5 cm) for an adult and about one-third the depth of the chest for a child.
f. Give 30 compressions (at a rate of 100 to 120 compressions per minute).
g. Push smoothly.
h. Allow the chest to fully recoil after each compression.

Skill Sheet 2-1 Adult and Child CPR *(continued)*

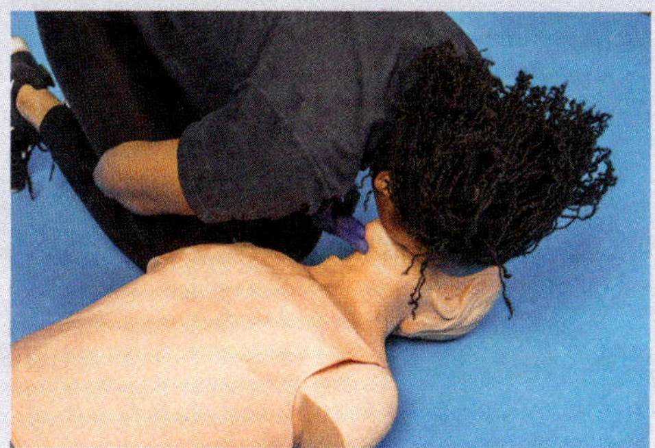

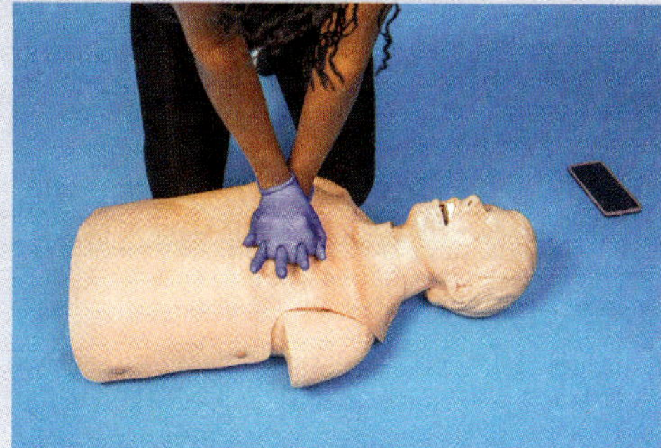

6 **B = Breaths.**
Give two rescue breaths while keeping the person's airway open, using a mouth-to-barrier device when possible:

a. Pinch the person's nose shut and make a tight seal with your mouth on the mouth-to-barrier device or the person's mouth. If unwilling or unable to give rescue breaths, give compression-only CPR instead.
b. Give two rescue breaths, each lasting 1 second and with just enough force for the chest to rise. Take a normal breath for yourself after each rescue breath.
c. Watch for chest rise to determine if your rescue breaths go in.
d. Allow for chest deflation after each rescue breath.
e. If you see chest rise after the 2 rescue breaths, give 30 chest compressions.
f. If the first rescue breath does not make the chest rise, retilt the person's head and give a second rescue breath. If the second rescue breath does not make the chest rise, assume an airway obstruction and follow the steps for treating an unresponsive person with an airway obstruction (p. 34).

7 Continue sets of 30 chest compressions and 2 rescue breaths until an AED or EMS arrives, or until the person begins breathing or moving. AED use is discussed in Chapter 3. If a bystander is present, they could help by giving chest compressions while you perform rescue breathing, or vice versa.

Compression-Only CPR

Compression-only CPR, or hands-only CPR, is CPR without rescue breaths. It is easy to teach, remember, and perform when compared with conventional CPR. It encourages bystanders help someone in a cardiac emergency, especially if the bystander is untrained, unable, or unwilling to give rescue breaths.

To perform compression-only CPR, follow the steps previously outlined in the RAB-CAB mnemonic up to C = *Compressions* and continue providing compressions until EMS arrives.

FYI

Chest Compressions

Effective chest compressions require significant effort on the part of the rescuer. It is physically exhausting to perform compressions, and compressions performed too lightly will not adequately pump the heart.

This is why multirescuer CPR includes rotating between providing rescue breaths and providing compressions, to allow the compressor to rest and maintain strong compressive force.

Infant CPR

CPR for infants (younger than 1 year) follows the same RAB-CAB format as for adults and children, but with some key differences in technique. First, the proper techniques for providing chest compressions are the two-thumbs technique (also referred to as the encircling hands technique) or, if you are unable to fit your hands around the infant, the heel-of-one-hand technique. Second, the compression depth is much less.

To perform CPR on an infant, follow the steps in **SKILL SHEET 2-2**.

FYI

Infant Compression Techniques

The two-finger compression technique (with the index and middle fingers compressing the center of the chest) is no longer recommended for infants due to ineffectiveness in achieving proper depth. New CPR guidelines recommend either the two-thumbs technique or the heel-of-one-hand technique as shown in Skill Sheet 2-2.

Infectious Diseases and Cardiac Arrest

A person can become infected from respiratory droplets when an infected person coughs, sneezes, or speaks. Infectious diseases may also be spread by touching a contaminated surface or object, and then touching your mouth, nose, eyes, or face.

This presents a dilemma for a CPR provider who is concerned about compromising their own health and perhaps life, yet wants to give CPR as an attempt to save the life of a person in cardiac arrest. If an adult, child, or infant who is known to have an infectious disease is in cardiac arrest, perform compression-only CPR as described previously, with two additions: (1) Cover the person's nose and mouth with a cloth or face mask and (2) Cover your nose and mouth with a face mask (see pp. 5–6) or cloth.

Skill Sheet 2-2 Infant CPR

Note: Whenever possible, use a mouth-to-barrier device to prevent disease transmission. Always take standard precautions.

Use the **RAB-CAB** mnemonic to remember what to do.

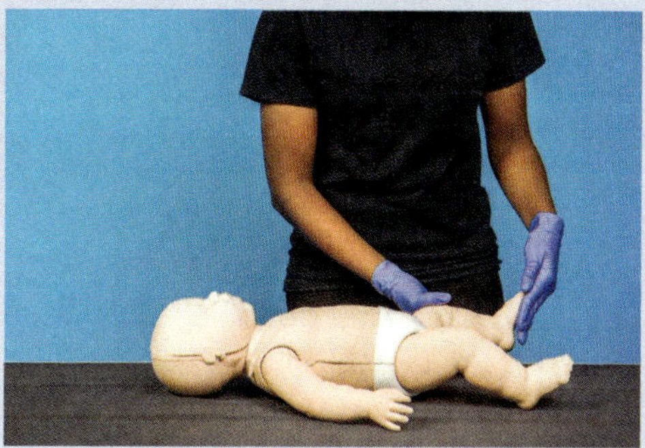

1 R = Responsive?

Tap the bottom of the infant's foot and shout their name.

a. If the infant moves, cries, or reacts, they are responsive. Continue first aid.
b. If the infant does not move, cry, or react, they are unresponsive. Continue to the next step, *A = Activate EMS and get an AED.*

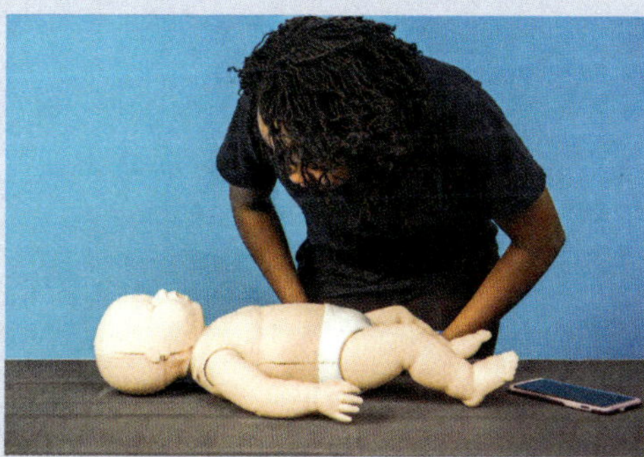

3 B = Breathing?

Take 5 to 10 seconds to check for breathing or only gasping by observing the infant from the neck to waist for movement (rise and fall). If the infant is not breathing or only gasping, continue to the next step, *C = Compressions*. CPR providers should not check for a pulse.

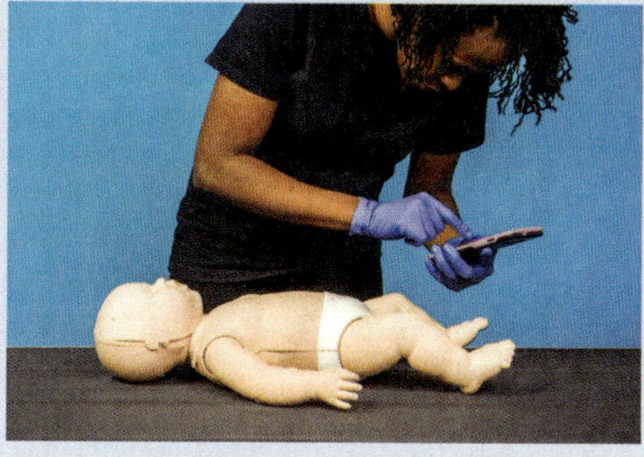

2 A = Activate EMS and get an AED.

a. Shout for nearby help.
b. If someone responds, have them call 9-1-1, set the phone to speaker mode, and get an AED while you start CPR. If a phone is not available, have them leave to call 9-1-1 and get an AED while you start CPR.
c. If no one responds and you are alone, perform CPR for 5 sets (30 chest compressions and 2 rescue breaths per set), call 9-1-1 and then get an AED. **DO NOT** call 9-1-1 until after 5 sets of CPR.

(continues)

Skill Sheet 2-2 Infant CPR

(continued)

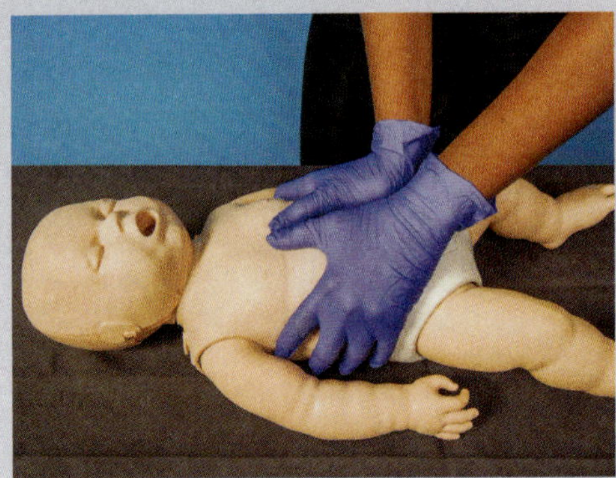

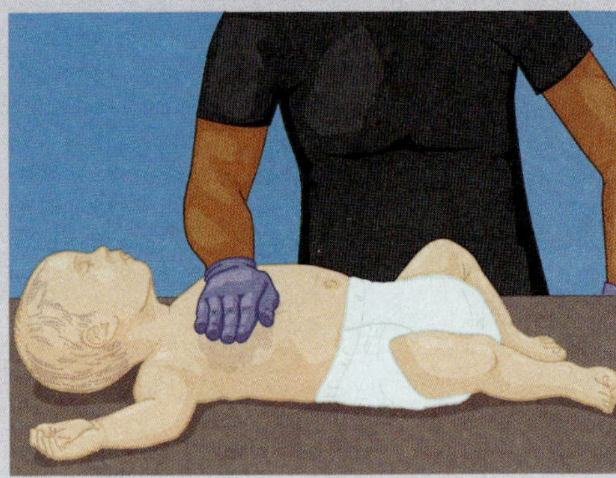

4 **C = Compressions.**

Place the infant faceup on a flat, firm surface. If possible, use an elevated surface (eg, table, cabinet top). Use the two-thumbs (encircling hands) technique to provide compressions. If you are unable to fit your hands around the infant or can't push hard enough with two thumbs, use the heel-of-one-hand technique. Any pausing during compressions should be less than 10 seconds. If the CPR provider is unable or unwilling to give rescue breaths, give compression-only CPR.

4a. ***Two Thumbs (Encircling Hands) Technique (left photo):***

a. Place both thumbs on the lower third of the breastbone (sternum) with both touching the imaginary nipple line and the fingers encircling around the infant's back and chest.

b. Give 30 chest compressions:
   - Push hard: about 1.5 inches (4 cm) straight down (at least one-third of the chest's diameter).
   - Push fast (100 to 120 compressions per minute).
   - At the end of each compression, let the infant's chest come back up to its normal position.

4b. ***Heel-of-One-Hand Technique (right image):***

a. Place the heel of one hand on the center of the infant's chest, on the imaginary nipple line. Keep your fingers raised and off the chest.

b. Give 30 chest compressions:
   - Push hard: about 1.5 inches (4 cm) straight downward (at least one-third of the chest's diameter).
   - Push fast (100 to 120 compressions per minute).
   - At the end of each compression, let the infant's chest come back up to its normal position.

Skill Sheet 2-2 Infant CPR

(continued)

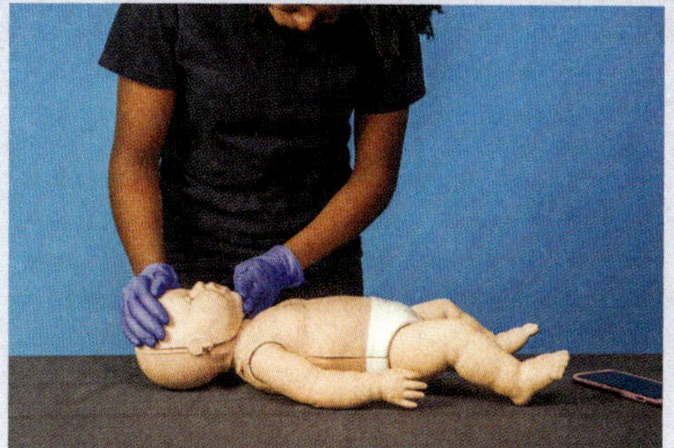

5 **A = Airway.**
Open the infant's airway using the head tilt–chin lift maneuver. **DO NOT** tilt the head back too far (tilt only to a neutral position). For a suspected neck injury, use the jaw-thrust maneuver without tilting the head (see p.15). If the jaw thrust does not open the airway, gently use the head tilt–chin lift maneuver. The infant will die without an open airway.

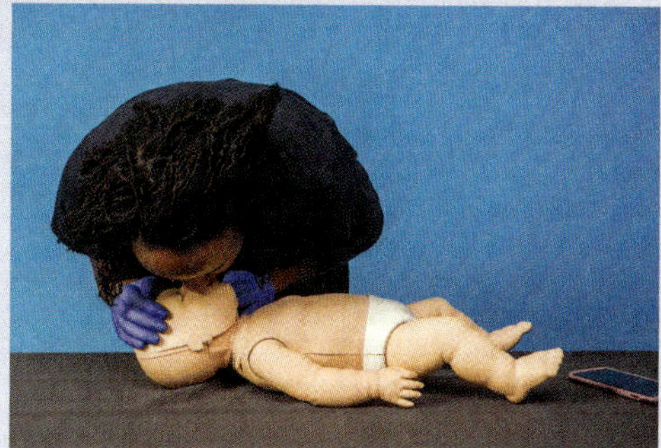

6 **B = Breaths.**

a. Cover the infant's mouth with a mouth-to-barrier device if possible. If not possible, cover the infant's mouth and nose with your mouth and make an airtight seal. If this does not work, try either mouth-to-mouth or mouth-to-nose rescue breaths.
b. Give 2 rescue breaths, each lasting 1 second, just enough to make the infant's chest rise.
c. Take a normal breath for yourself between each rescue breath.
d. Continue CPR until one of the following occurs:
   - The infant begins breathing.
   - EMS arrives and takes over.
   - You become physically exhausted and are unable to continue.
e. If another person is available, trade off about every 5 sets of CPR (2 minutes).

CPR Performance Mistakes

Mistakes made while performing CPR can usually be placed into one of these two categories:

1. Rescue breathing mistakes
   - Failing to ensure the airway is open
   - Failing to pinch the nose shut in a child and adult or not covering mouth and nose in an infant
   - Providing rescue breaths that are too fast or too forceful
   - Failing to watch the person's chest rise and fall
   - Failing to maintain a tight seal around the mouth, pocket mask, or barrier device
   - Using outdated rescue breathing techniques

2. Chest compression mistakes
   - Pivoting at knees instead of hips (eg, rocking motion) when giving adult or child compressions
   - Using the wrong compression site (eg, too high or too low on the chest)
   - Bending elbows (arms should be kept straight with elbows locked)
   - Failing to place shoulders above sternum (arms should be vertical)
   - Touching your fingers to the person's chest when giving adult or child compressions
   - Providing quick, stabbing compressions
   - Interruptions in compressions for greater than 5 seconds
   - Failing to allow the chest to fully recoil (eg, leaning on the chest)
   - Failing to keep your hand in contact with the person's chest between each compression (some instructors teach to lift hands off the chest, which allows the chest to recoil, but this could lead to stabbing compressions)
   - Using outdated compression techniques

When Not to Start CPR

Generally speaking, CPR should be initiated on all persons who are unresponsive and not breathing (or only gasping). However, there are a few situations in which CPR should not be started:

- Scene is unsafe
- Obviously fatal injuries (eg, decapitation)
- Airway is obstructed with ice (ie, in mouth and throat)
- Chest is frozen stiff and cannot be compressed

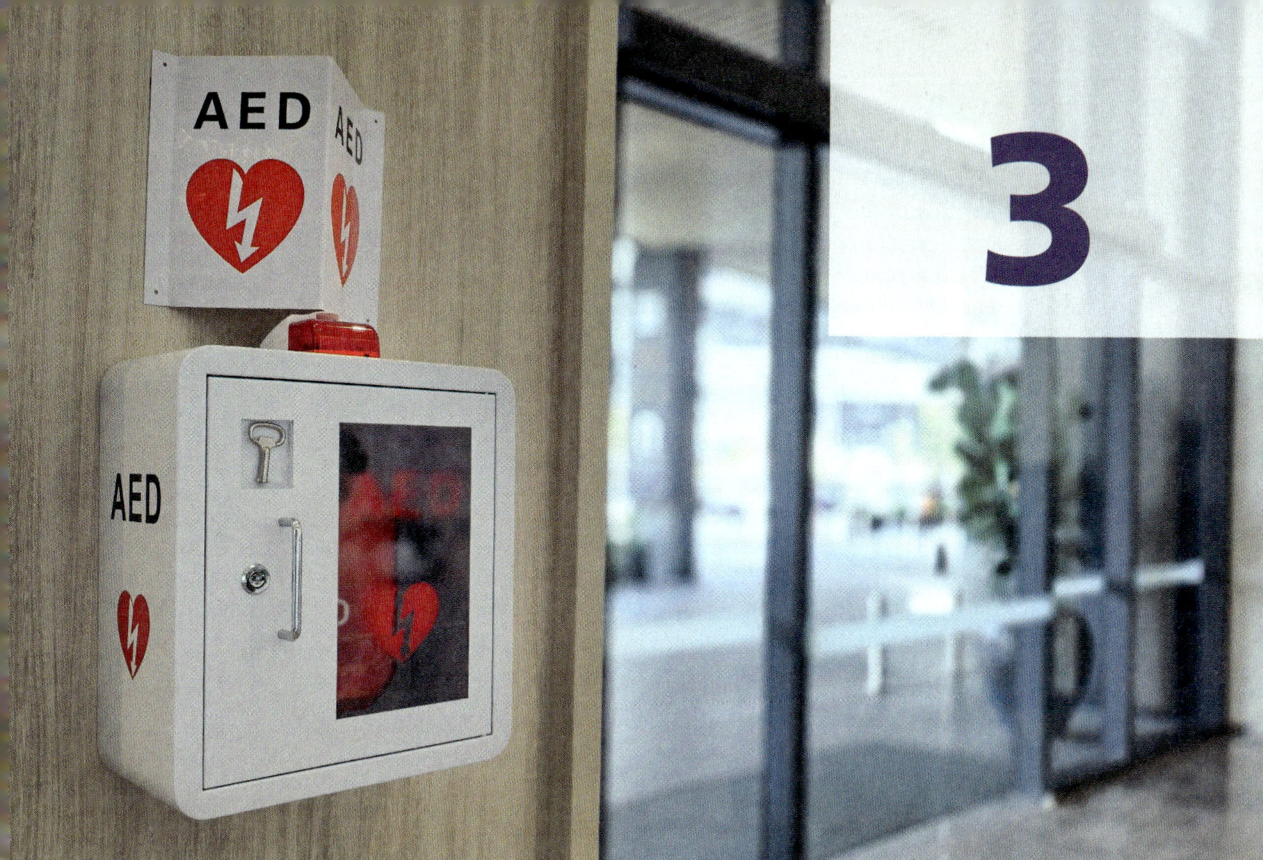

© ThamKC/Shutterstock

Automated External Defibrillation

CHAPTER AT A GLANCE

Automated External Defibrillators

More than 70% of all out-of-hospital cardiac arrests involve one of two irregular electrical heart rhythms (heartbeats). The first, ventricular fibrillation, is when the heart's ventricles (bottom two chambers of the heart) quiver or twitch and do not produce effective heartbeats. The second is ventricular tachycardia, in which the heart beats so rapidly that it cannot fill with blood between beats. Essentially, in both conditions, not enough blood is pumped from the heart, which results in a type of cardiac arrest.

An automated external defibrillator, or AED, analyzes the heart rhythm to determine if an electric shock, or defibrillation, is necessary. If it is, the AED will prompt the rescuer to deliver the shock to the heart of a person in cardiac arrest. The purpose of this shock is to correct an abnormal electrical disturbance and reestablish a heart rhythm that will result in normal electrical and pumping function. Using an AED as soon as possible increases the person's chance of survival.

Many different AED models exist. The principles for use are the same for each, but the displays, controls, and options vary slightly. The AED is attached to a cable connected to two adhesive pads (electrodes) that are placed on the person's chest. The pad and cable system send the electrical signal from the heart into the device for rhythm analysis and alert the rescuer to deliver the electric shock to the person when needed. Most have voice prompts or visual displays that guide users through each step. This intuitive system enables anyone to deliver defibrillation with minimal training.

Using an AED

Once you have determined the need for the AED (person unresponsive and not breathing), the basic operation of all AED models follows the sequence in **SKILL SHEET 3-1**.

1. Some AEDs power on by pressing an On/Off button. Others power on when the AED case lid is opened. Once the power is on, the AED will quickly go through some internal checks and will then begin to provide voice and/or screen prompts.
2. Expose the person's chest. The skin must be fairly dry so that the pads will adhere and conduct electricity properly. If necessary, dry the skin with a towel. Because an adult's excessive chest hair may also interfere with adhesion and electrical conduction, you may need to quickly shave the area where the pads are to be placed. Razors are often included in AED cases.
3. Apply the AED pads.
   a. For an adult or large child, remove the backing from the pads and apply them firmly to the person's bare chest according to the diagram on the pads (**FIGURE 3-1A**). One pad is placed to the right of the person's breastbone, just below the collarbone and above the right nipple. The second pad is placed on the person's left side of the chest, left of the nipple and above the lower rib margin. For an adult wearing a bra, adjust its position only as much as necessary, such as moving the straps, instead of removing it. The pads should only touch skin.
   b. For an infant or small child: Check to see if pediatric equipment is available, such as a pediatric attenuator device (reduces the energy of an electric shock to a level that is safe for a child) or pediatric pads. If pediatric equipment is not available, use the adult equipment. Avoid having the pads touch each other by placing one pad in the middle of the chest and the other pad on the back, between the shoulder blades (**FIGURE 3-1B**).
4. Make sure the cable is attached to the AED and verify that no one is in contact with the person. Stand clear for analysis of the heart's electrical activity.
5. If no shock is advised, resume CPR and follow the prompts.
6. The AED will alert you to push a button to administer the shock if one is advised. Confirm that no one is touching the person, then follow the instructions from the AED. Begin CPR immediately following the shock, and follow the prompts, which will include reanalyzing the heart rhythm (about every 5 sets of CPR [approximately 2 minutes]). If the shock successfully corrected the irregular heartbeat, the person will begin to breathe or move. Assess the breathing and place the person into the recovery position (**FIGURE 3-2**) to keep the airway clear. Continue providing care until EMS arrives and takes over.

Skill Sheet 3-1 Using an AED

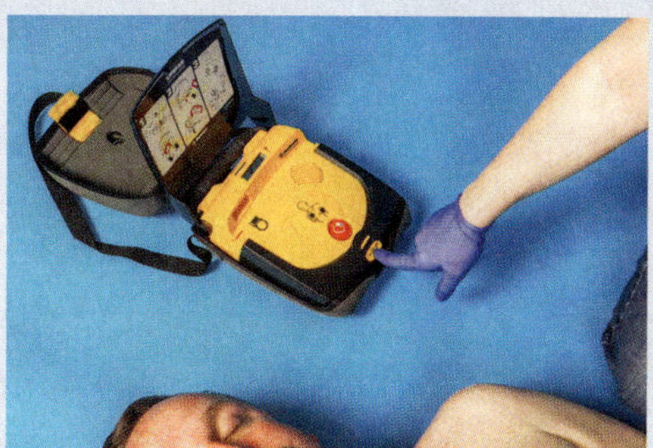

1 Turn on the AED.

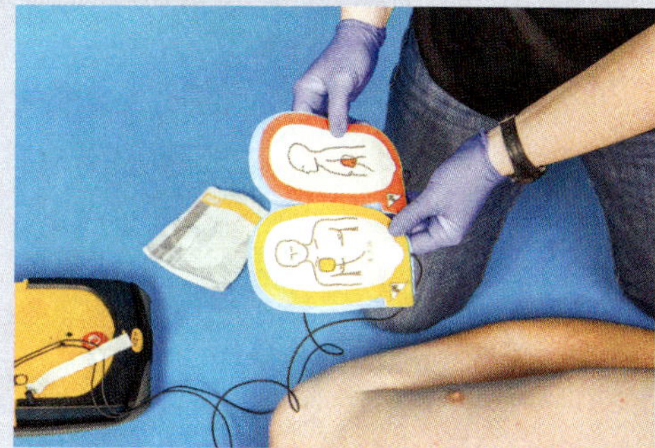

2 Attach the pads to the person's bare, dry chest (as shown on the pads). If needed, plug the cables into the AED. For children and infants, keep pads separated with one pad on the center of the chest and the second pad centered on the back.

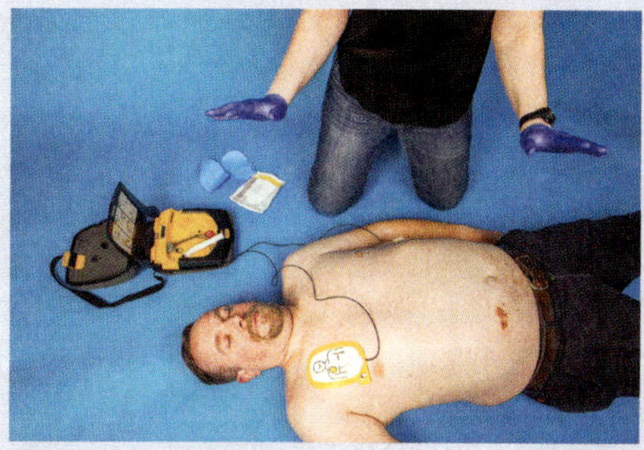

3 Stay clear of the person. Make sure no one, including yourself, is touching the person. Say, "Clear!"

4 Allow the AED to analyze the heart. The AED will prompt one of two actions:

a. If a shock is advised, stay clear and press the Shock button.

b. If no shock is advised, do not provide a shock, but leave the pads in place.

5 Whether or not a shock is provided, give 5 sets of CPR (approximately 2 minutes) unless the person moves, begins to breathe, or wakes up. Even if the person wakes up, leave the AED pads on until EMS arrives.

6 Repeat Steps 4–5 until the person moves or begins to breathe, or until EMS takes over.

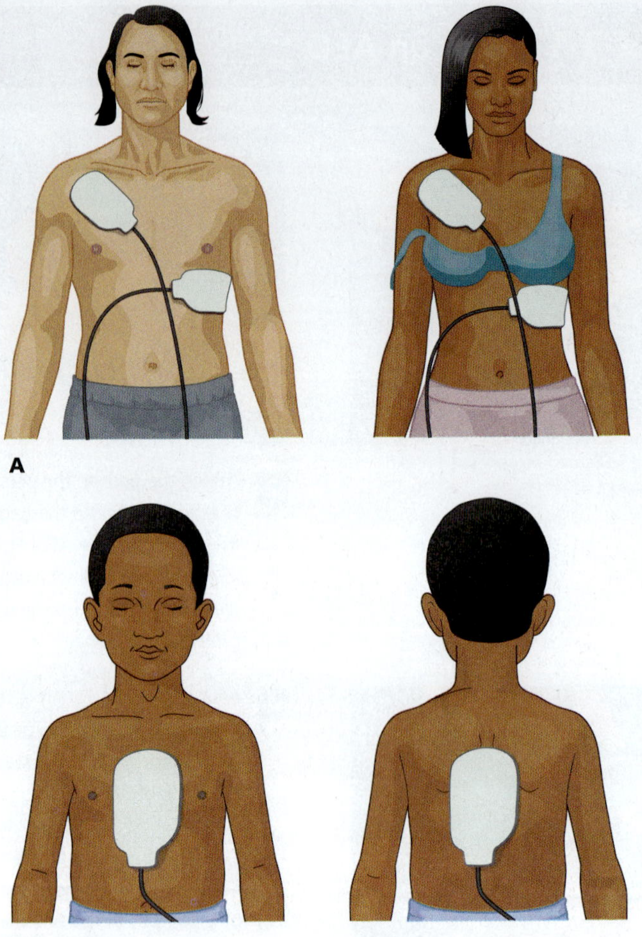

FIGURE 3-1 Proper AED pad placement. **A.** Adults. **B.** Children and infants.

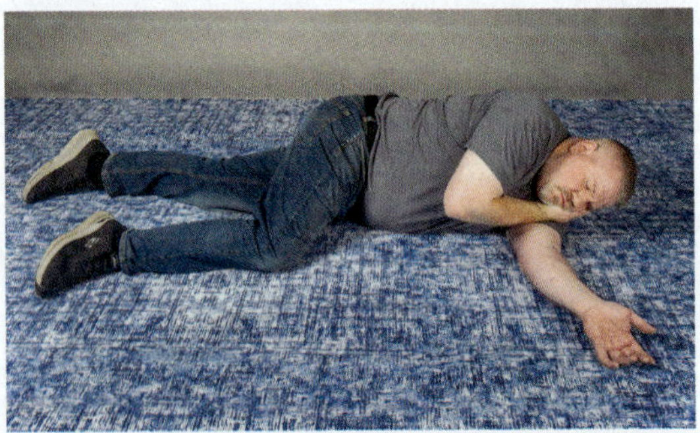

FIGURE 3-2 The recovery position uses gravity to keep the airway open and allow fluids to drain out of the nose and mouth (instead of into the throat).

AED Special Considerations

What to Look For	What to Do
Wet skin, lying in shallow water, or on snow	■ Move the person out of the water or off the snow. ■ Wipe the chest dry before attaching the pads.
Chest hair	Remove hair if it may prevent the pads from sticking to the skin. Do this by either: ■ Shaving the area where pads will be placed. The AED's case should contain a razor to use, or ■ Apply adhesive tape (eg, duct, masking, bandage) firmly onto the hair and rip the tape off. It may be necessary to repeat this several times. **DO NOT** use the AED pads to rip out hair.
Bra or other undergarment	Adjust its position only as much as necessary, such as moving the straps, instead of removing it. AED pads should only touch skin.
Medication patches (eg, nitroglycerin, nicotine, pain medication)	■ While wearing gloves, or using a cloth or paper towel, remove the patch. ■ **DO NOT** place an AED pad over a medicine patch.
Implanted devices (pacemaker or defibrillator)	Move the pad at least 2 inches (5 cm) away from the device. **DO NOT** place an AED pad directly over the implanted device.
Child or infant	The procedure is the same as for an adult. Some AEDs may have pediatric equipment, such as a pediatric attenuator device (reduces the energy of an electric shock to a level that is safe for a child) or pediatric pads (**FIGURE 3-3**). If pediatric equipment is not available, use the adult equipment. Avoid having the pads touch each other by placing one pad in the middle of the chest and the other pad on the back, between the shoulder blades.

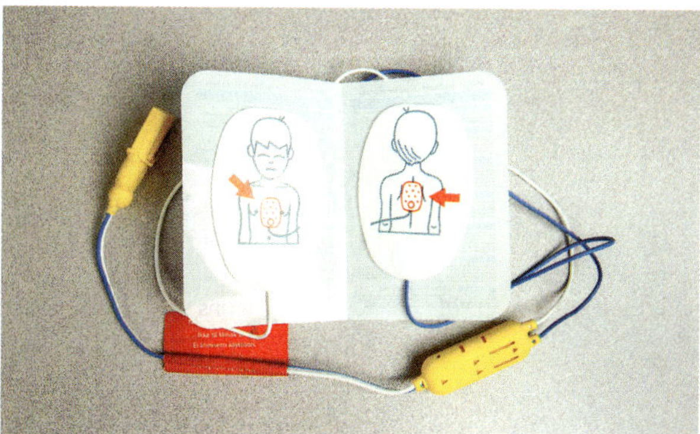

FIGURE 3-3 Pediatric AED pads with pediatric dose attenuator (yellow).

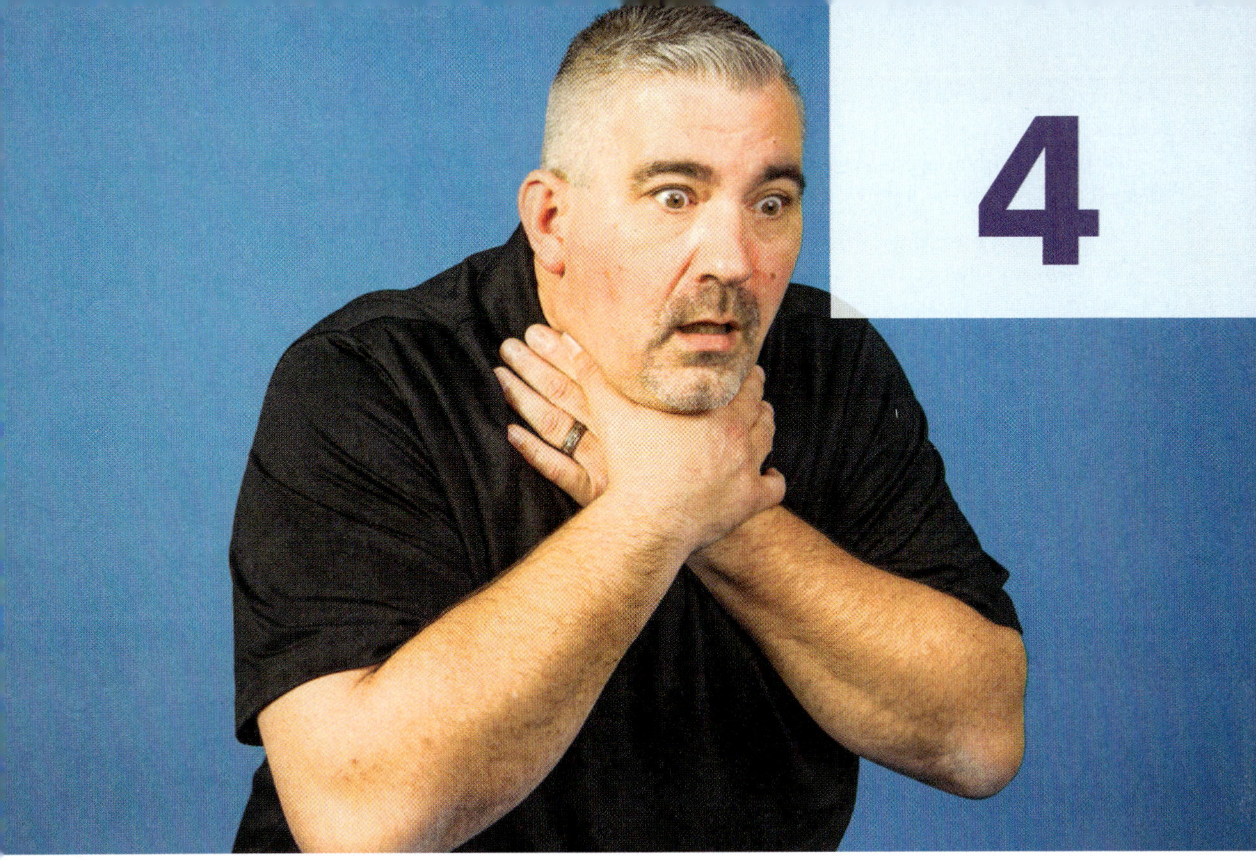

Airway Obstruction

Recognizing Airway Obstruction

People can choke on all types of objects. Foods such as candy, peanuts, and grapes are major offenders because of their shapes and consistencies. Nonfood choking deaths are often caused by balloons, balls, marbles, toys, and coins inhaled by children and infants.

An object lodged in the airway can cause a mild or severe airway obstruction. In a mild airway obstruction, good air exchange is present and the person is able to make forceful coughing efforts in an attempt to relieve the obstruction. The person should be encouraged to cough. If coughing does not clear the obstruction quickly, activate EMS, monitor the person's condition, and intervene if signs of a severe obstruction develop.

CHAPTER AT A GLANCE

A person with a severe airway obstruction will have poor air exchange. The signs of a severe airway obstruction include the following:

- Increased breathing difficulty
- Weak and ineffective cough
- Inability to speak or breathe
- Skin, fingernail beds, inside of mouth, or lips turn blue or gray

The person who is choking may also appear panicky and desperate and may clutch at their throat to communicate that they are choking. This motion is known as the universal distress signal for choking (**FIGURE 4-1**).

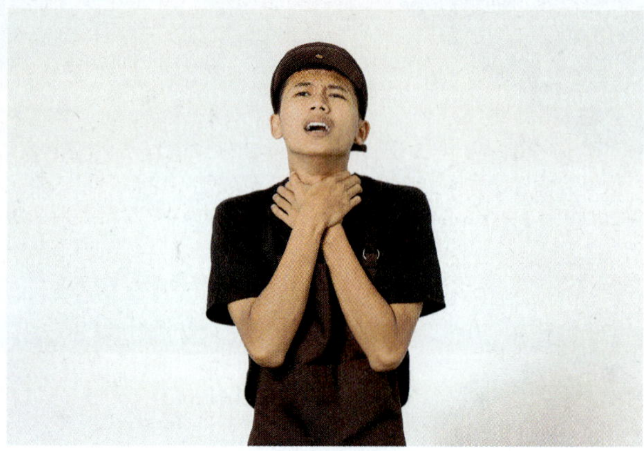

FIGURE 4-1 Universal sign for choking.

Caring for Airway Obstruction

Adult and Child Airway Obstruction

If . . .	Then . . .
The person is responsive and shows signs of mild airway obstruction (choking): ▪ Good air exchange is present. ▪ Able to make forceful coughing efforts in an attempt to relieve the obstruction	▪ Encourage continued coughing, but otherwise do not intervene. Aggressive treatment (eg, back blows, abdominal thrusts, chest compressions) may cause complications and could worsen the airway obstruction. ▪ Monitor the person until they improve. If there is no improvement in a couple of minutes, call 9-1-1 because a severe airway obstruction can occur at any time.
The person is responsive and shows signs of complete airway obstruction: ▪ Difficulty breathing ▪ Unable to cough forcefully	1. **DO NOT** ask them if they are okay. Instead, ask them if they are choking and if you can help them. If they nod "yes," tell them you are going to help. 2. Have someone call 9-1-1.

<table>
<tr><th>If . . .</th><th>Then . . .</th></tr>
<tr><td>

- Unable to talk
- Skin, fingernail beds, or lips turn blue or gray
- Appears panicky and desperate
- Points to their mouth or grasps at their throat

Note: It is important to distinguish choking from fainting, heart attack, seizure, anaphylaxis, and other conditions that may cause sudden respiratory distress or loss of responsiveness.

</td><td>

3. Give back blows (**SKILL SHEET 4-1**):
   a. Stand to the side and slightly behind the choking person. If they are a child or in a wheelchair, kneel behind them.
   b. Support the person by reaching your arm either over their arm or under their armpit and placing it diagonally across the person's chest. Place the palm of that hand on the person's upper chest or shoulder. **DO NOT** keep the person in an upright or vertical position. If they are not bending over when the jolt of the back blow dislodges the object, the object may become stuck deeper in the airway.
   c. Give five hard back blows with the heel of the hand that is not supporting the person. Aim for the area in between their shoulder blades. **DO NOT** just pat them on the back; use hard blows (eg, like driving or hitting a nail into a thick board with a hammer). Each blow should be a distinct effort to dislodge the obstruction.
   d. Quickly check after each back blow to see if the obstruction has been dislodged. The goal is to relieve the object with a blow, not to necessarily give all five back blows.

</td></tr>
<tr><td>The five back blows fail to dislodge the airway obstruction.</td><td>

Give abdominal thrusts (**SKILL SHEET 4-2**):

1. Stand behind the person or kneel behind a child or person in a wheelchair. If the person is significantly taller than you, have them kneel or sit.
2. Put one foot in front of the other foot; this provides stability during the thrusts and if the person becomes unresponsive and collapses, they can slide down your leg to the ground or floor.
3. Wrap your arms around the person's waist. Locate the person's navel (belly button) using two fingers (right-handed people will usually use their left hand). If your arms cannot encircle the person's waist (eg, pregnant woman, or a very large person and you are smaller than them), use chest thrusts (discussed later).
4. Make a fist with the other hand (right-handed people will usually use their right hand to make a fist). Place the thumb side of the fist just above the person's navel and below the tip of the breastbone (sternum). Grab the fist with the first hand.
5. Give up to five abdominal thrusts by quickly pulling the fist inward and upward into the person's abdomen. Each thrust should be a separate and distinct effort to dislodge the object.

</td></tr>
<tr><td>The obstruction does not get dislodged and is still in place.</td><td>

Repeat alternating between back blows and abdominal thrusts until one or more of the following occurs:

- The person can cough forcefully, breathe, or speak.
- The person becomes unresponsive.
- EMS or someone with training takes over.

</td></tr>
</table>

If . . .	Then . . .
The person becomes unresponsive.	▪ Support the person while carefully lowering them to the ground. ▪ If EMS has not arrived or has not been called, call them immediately. ▪ Begin CPR, starting with chest compressions. ▪ After each set of 30 compressions and before giving rescue breaths, open the mouth, look for an object in the back of the throat, and if seen, remove it.
The person is found unresponsive.	Follow the steps of CPR. ▪ If the person's chest does not rise when the first rescue breath is delivered, retilt the head and try again. If the second rescue breath does not result in chest rise, an object may be blocking the person's airway. ▪ After each set of 30 compressions and before giving rescue breaths, open the mouth, look for an object in the back of the throat, and if seen, remove it. **DO NOT** use blind finger sweeps in people with an airway obstruction.
Solid material or an object can be seen in the airway.	Remove the solid material or object only if seen. **DO NOT** use a blind finger sweep.
The person is pregnant, in a wheelchair, or very large, or you are small.	Provide chest thrusts (**FIGURE 4-2**): **1.** Position yourself behind the person. A choking person who is large or tall may need to kneel in front of you. **2.** Put your arms under the person's armpits and make a fist with one hand (right-handed people will usually use their right hand). Place the thumb side of your fist on the lower half of the breastbone (sternum). Grab the fist with your other hand. **3.** Pull your hands quickly back into the chest. This is similar to abdominal thrusts, except pull straight back instead of upward. **4.** If the person becomes unresponsive, move them to a flat, firm surface and begin chest compressions.
The object has been dislodged and the person has a persistent cough or feels something is stuck in their throat.	Seek professional medical care because injuries may have occurred.

Self-Administering Abdominal Thrusts

If you are alone and choking, call 9-1-1 and stay on the line. You will not be able to speak, but the dispatcher may be able to trace your call and send help if you lose consciousness. Then, perform abdominal thrusts on yourself.

First, locate a steady, hard surface such as a countertop or chair without wheels. Place a hand flat just under your breastbone to protect it. Then, fall onto the object, striking below your hand (**FIGURE 4-3**). Continue until object is dislodged. Then, talk to the 9-1-1 dispatcher.

If a hard surface is not available, give yourself abdominal thrusts with your hands. Locate your navel with your index and middle fingers. With your free hand, make a fist and place the thumb side against your stomach above the two fingers. Remove the two fingers and use that hand to grasp the fist. Pull the fist inward and upward in quick motions, as you would on someone else. If you are pregnant, position your hands over your chest instead and pull inward. Continue until the object is dislodged. Then, talk to the 9-1-1 dispatcher.

Skill Sheet 4-1 Adult or Child Choking: Back Blows

Note: Always take standard precautions.

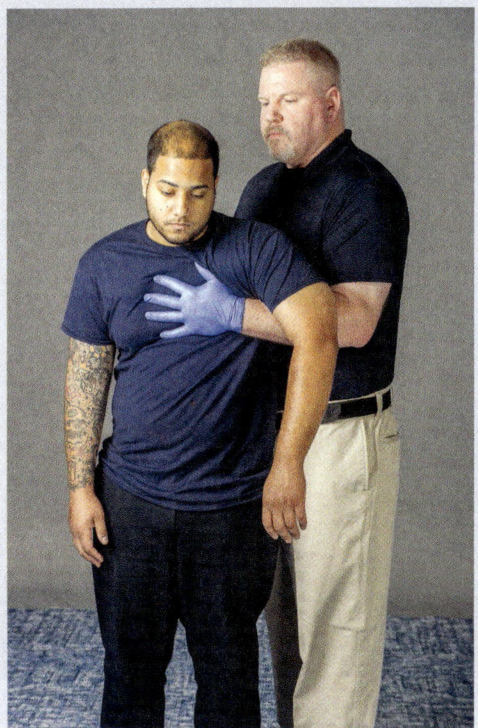

1 Stand behind the person and slightly to one side. If they are a child or in a wheelchair, or if you are very tall, kneel behind them. Support the person by reaching one of your arms either over their arm or under their armpit and placing it diagonally across the person's chest. Place the palm of that hand on the person's upper chest or shoulder. Leave your other hand free.

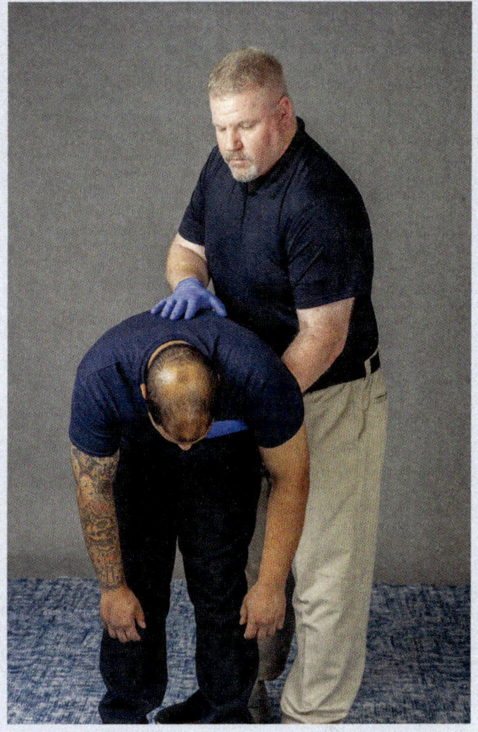

2 Have the person bend over at the waist. **DO NOT** keep them in an upright or a vertical position. If they are not bending over when the jolt of the back blow dislodges the object, the dislodged object may become stuck deeper in the airway.

(*continues*)

Skill Sheet 4-1 Adult or Child Choking: Back Blows *(continued)*

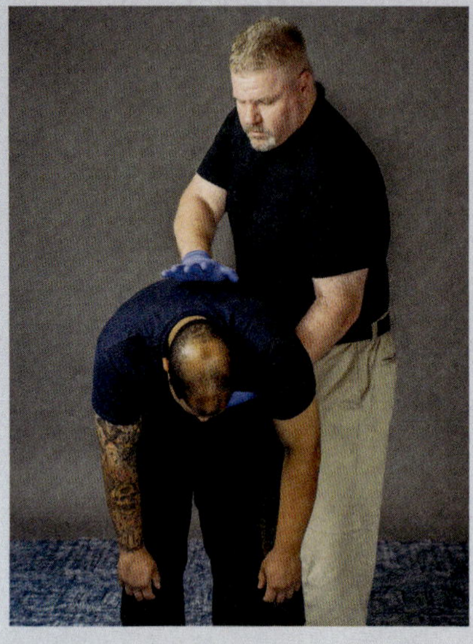

3 With your fingertips up, use the heel of your free hand to firmly strike the person between their shoulder blades. Each blow should be a distinct effort to dislodge the object.

4 If five back blows do not dislodge the object, give up to five abdominal thrusts (see Skill Sheet 4-2).

Skill Sheet 4-2 Adult or Child Choking: Abdominal Thrusts

Note: Always take standard precautions.

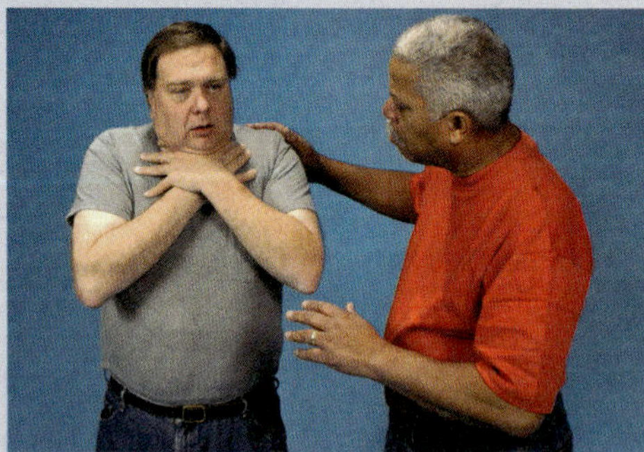

1 If the five back blows do not dislodge the object or the person is still unable to speak (see Skill Sheet 4-1), give up to five abdominal thrusts. Do this by following the remaining steps.

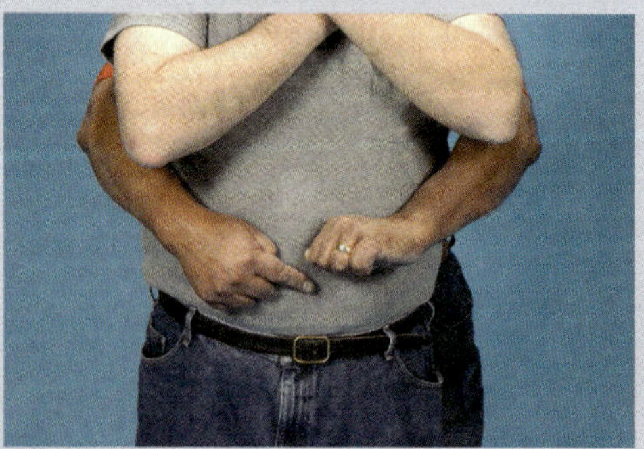

2 Assist the person into an upright position. Use two fingers to locate the person's navel. Keeping your fingers on the navel, move behind the person. Stand behind an adult; stand or kneel behind a child. Wrap your arms around the person's waist.

Skill Sheet 4-2 Adult or Child Choking: Abdominal Thrusts

(continued)

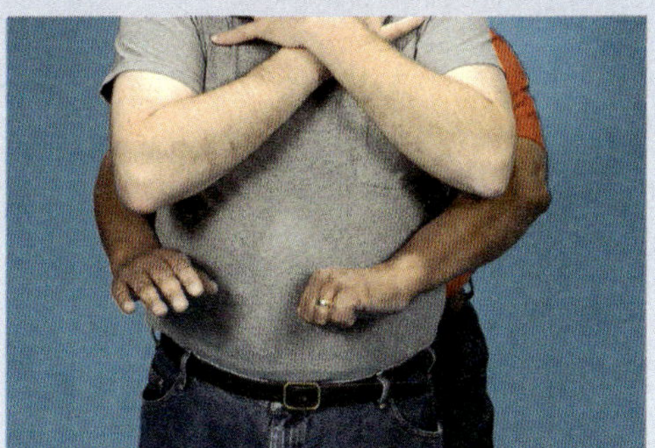

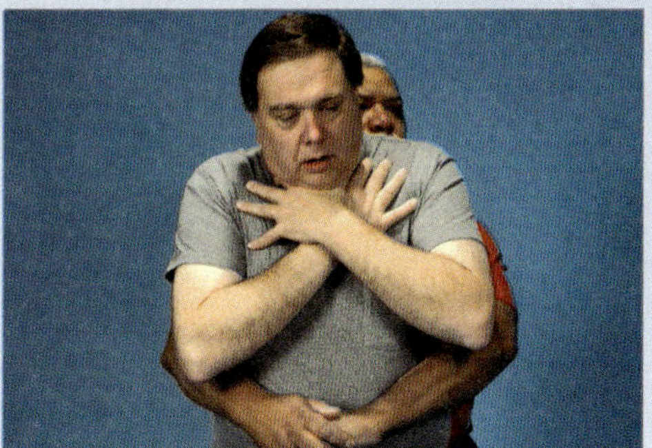

3 Make a fist with your hand and place the thumb side of the fist against the person's stomach, just above your two fingers (above the person's navel and below the tip of the breastbone [sternum]).

4 Remove the two fingers and use that hand to grasp the fist. Thrust the fist into the person's abdomen with a quick upward motion. Each thrust should be a separate and distinct effort to dislodge the object. After each thrust, quickly determine if the abdominal thrust dislodged the object. The goal is to relieve the object with a thrust, not to necessarily give all five abdominal thrusts before checking.

5 If the five abdominal thrusts do not dislodge the object, repeat a combination of five back blows and five abdominal thrusts until one of the following occurs:

- The object is dislodged and the person starts breathing.
- EMS or a person with training arrives and takes over.
- Another person arrives and allows you to take turns giving back blows and abdominal thrusts.
- The person becomes unresponsive and collapses to the ground or floor.

6 If the person becomes unresponsive, gently lower them to the ground and place them faceup. Look in the back of the throat for an object and, if seen, remove it; if not, begin CPR:

a. Give 30 chest compressions.
b. Give two rescue breaths. If the first rescue breath does not cause the chest to rise, retilt the head and attempt a second breath.
c. If the second rescue breath still does not result in chest rise, continue sets of 30 chest compressions and two rescue breaths. Each time before giving the first of the two rescue breaths, look into the mouth for an object; if seen, remove it.

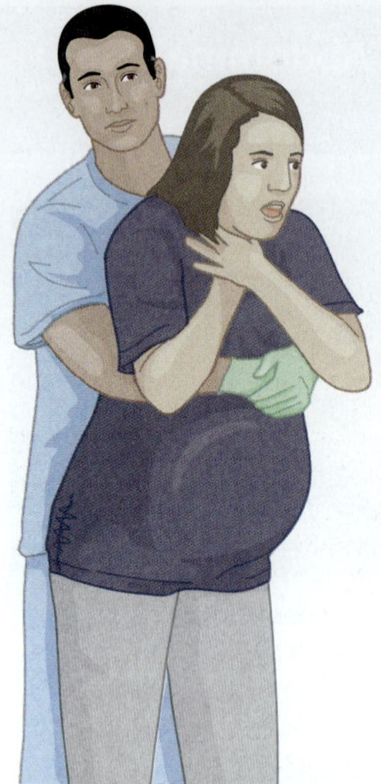

FIGURE 4-2 Chest thrusts are similar to CPR chest compressions, but are sharper and delivered at a slower rate, and the choking person is standing. Hands are placed on the lower half of the breastbone (sternum).

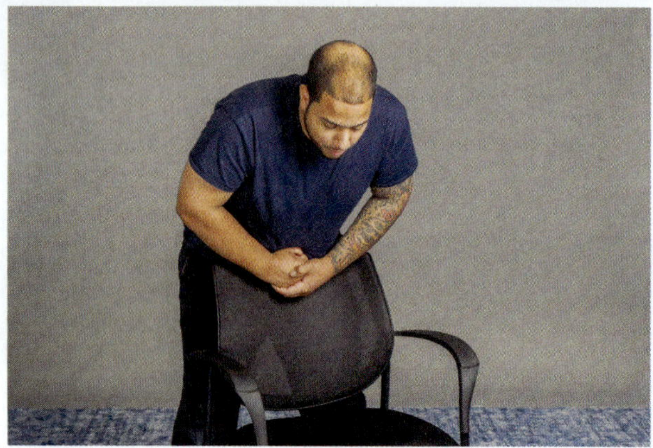

FIGURE 4-3 Self-administering abdominal thrusts over a chair without wheels.

Infant Airway Obstruction

For a responsive infant with an airway obstruction, give five back blows and five chest thrusts instead of abdominal thrusts to relieve the obstruction:

1. Support the infant's head and neck and lay the infant facedown on your forearm, then lower your arm holding the infant onto your thigh.
2. Give five back blows between the infant's shoulder blades with the heel of your hand.
3. While supporting the back of the infant's head, roll the infant faceup onto the other arm, and brace that arm against your other thigh. Using the heel-of-the-hand positioning for CPR, give five chest thrusts, 1 second apart. Note that these are separate and distinct thrusts and are not like the faster CPR compressions. Keep your fingers raised and push straight downward with the heel of your hand. **DO NOT** give CPR compressions; thrust upward toward the head, or use the two-finger technique.
4. Repeat these steps until the object is removed or the infant becomes unresponsive.

For an infant with an airway obstruction, follow the steps in **SKILL SHEET 4-3**.

Skill Sheet 4-3 Infant Choking

Note: An infant is not breathing if they are unable to cry or make a sound. Always take standard precautions.

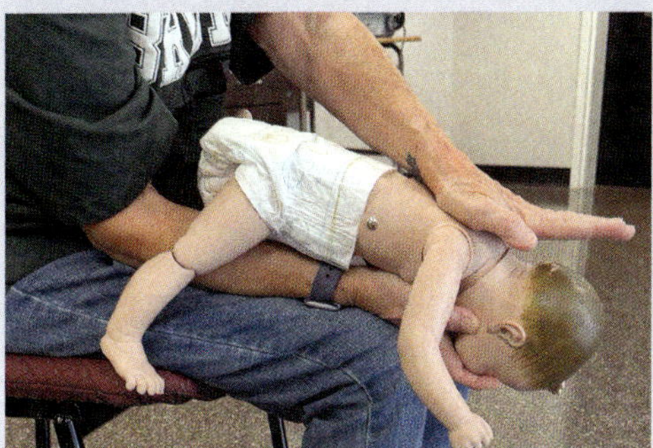

1 Give up to five separate and distinct back blows.

a. Sit down and place the infant's back along your forearm, cradling the back of the infant's head with your hand. Then, place your other arm along the infant's front, supporting the jaw with your thumb and fingers.

b. Turn the infant over so that they are facedown over your other forearm, with your hand supporting the jaw and the infant's head lower than their chest.

c. Brace your forearm and the infant against your thigh. (If holding the infant with your right hand and forearm, brace them against your right thigh; if using the left hand and arm, brace them against your left thigh.)

d. Give five back blows between the infant's shoulder blades with the heel of your free hand. Keep your fingers up to avoid hitting the infant's head or neck.

e. If the object does not come out, turn the infant onto their back while supporting the head.

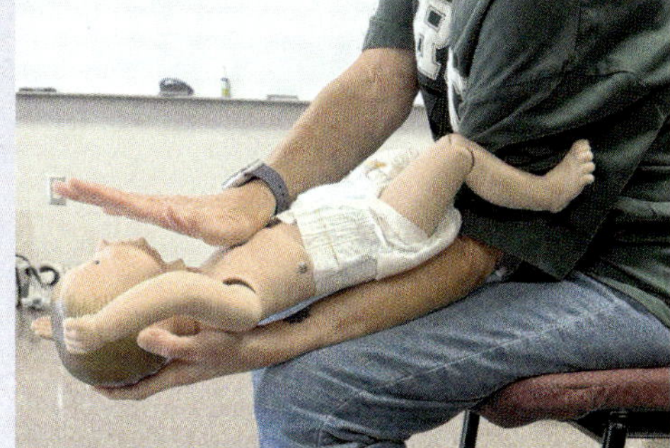

2 Give up to five separate and distinct chest thrusts.

a. Support the infant's head with your hand.

b. Lay the infant faceup over your forearm, tilt your arm down so the infant's head is lower than their chest.

c. Brace your forearm and the infant against your thigh, keeping their head lower than their body.

d. Place the heel of your free hand on the center of the infant's chest, just below the nipple line (this is the same location as for giving CPR compressions with the heel-of-the-hand technique). Keeping your fingers raised, push straight down into the chest with the heel of your hand.

e. Give the thrusts 1 second apart—this is not as fast as CPR compressions.

3 Continue alternating the five back blows and five chest thrusts without interruption until the infant breathes, coughs or cries, or until EMS or a trained person takes over.

4 If the infant becomes unresponsive, provide CPR:

a. Place the infant on a firm, flat surface.

b. Give 30 chest compressions.

c. Look into the infant's mouth for an object; if seen, remove it.

d. Give two rescue breaths.

e. Repeat Steps a–c until the object is dislodged and the infant begins to breathe, EMS arrives, or you become too exhausted to continue.

Courtesy of Rhonda Hunt.

Appendix A: CPR and AED Review

Using **TABLE A-1**, review the CPR and AED procedures using the RAB-CAB sequence.

TABLE A-1 Quick Review of CPR and AED Procedures Using the RAB-CAB Sequence

Steps/Action	Adults (at or past puberty)	Child (1 year to puberty)	Infant (younger than 1 year)
R = Responsive?			
Technique	Tap a shoulder and shout, "Are you okay?" An adult or child who is responsive will answer, move, or moan.		Tap the bottom of a foot and shout their name. A responsive infant will cry or move.
A = Activate EMS and get an AED. **(Shout for nearby help and call 9-1-1 or the emergency response number. An AED may or may not be available.)**			
When?	▪ If you are alone and do not have a phone, leave to call 9-1-1 and get an AED. When you return, apply the AED and follow the prompts. ▪ If another person is with you, send them to call and get an AED while you begin CPR immediately.	▪ If you are alone, and before calling 9-1-1, give 5 sets of 30 chest compressions and 2 rescue breaths (CPR). ▪ After 5 sets of CPR, call 9-1-1 and get an AED. ▪ When you return, apply the AED and follow the prompts.	
B = Breathing?			
▪ Place person faceup on a flat, firm surface. ▪ Observe from the neck to the waist for movement indicating breathing. Take 5 seconds but no more than 10 seconds.	If the person is not breathing or is only occasionally gasping (may sound like a quick inhalation or like a groan/snore), CPR is needed. If the person is breathing but not responding, CPR is not needed. If a spinal injury is not suspected, place the person in the recovery position to keep their airway clear. If a spinal injury is suspected, hold the person's head in alignment and keep it from moving. Monitor breathing.		
C = Chest compressions			
Where to place person?	Firm, flat surface (eg, floor, ground, sidewalk)		Can be placed on table or cabinet top

(continues)

TABLE A-1 Quick Review of CPR and AED Procedures Using the RAB-CAB Sequence (*continued*)

Steps/Action	Adults (at or past puberty)	Child (1 year to puberty)	Infant (younger than 1 year)
Where to place hands?	Center of chest and lower half of breastbone (sternum)		▪ Two-thumbs (encircling hands) technique: Both thumbs on lower third of the breastbone, both touching the imaginary nipple line and the fingers encircling the infant's back and chest OR ▪ Heel-of-one-hand technique, with the heel of the hand on the breastbone, below the nipple line
	Two hands: ▪ Heel of one hand on breastbone; other hand on top ▪ Fingers of both hands interlocked ▪ Arms straight with shoulders directly over the hands	Larger child: Same as for an adult Smaller child: Only heel of one hand	
Depth	At least 2 in. (5 cm) but no more than 2.4 in. (6 cm)	About 2 in. (5 cm) or one-third depth of the upper body (chest)	About 1.5 in. (4 cm) or one-third depth of the upper body (chest)
	DO NOT lean on the chest of an adult or child.		
	After each compression, allow full recoil of the chest.		
Rate	100 to 120 per minute (Follow the beat of the Bee Gees' song "Stayin' Alive," the beats from a smartphone application that was previously installed and is quickly accessible, or a dispatcher's directions heard over a cell phone's speaker.)		
Ratio of chest compressions to rescue breaths	30:2		

Steps/Action	Adults (at or past puberty)	Child (1 year to puberty)	Infant (younger than 1 year)
A = Airway open			
Technique	Head tilt–chin lift maneuver (if spinal injury is not suspected) Jaw-thrust maneuver (if spinal injury is suspected)		
B = Breaths			
Technique	▪ When possible, use a mouth-to-barrier device. If not possible, pinch the nose shut, and, with your mouth, make an airtight mouth-to-mouth seal. ▪ Give two rescue breaths: • Each rescue breath should last 1 second. • Blow just enough to make the chest rise. If first rescue breath does not cause chest to rise, retilt head and give second rescue breath. If second rescue breath does not make chest rise, the person's airway may be blocked by a foreign body. Continue CPR (30 compressions and 2 rescue breaths). Each time before giving a rescue breath, open the mouth and look for an object; if seen, remove it.		▪ Cover the infant's mouth and nose with your mouth, making an airtight seal. If this does not work, try either mouth-to-mouth or mouth-to-nose rescue breaths. ▪ Give two rescue breaths: • Each rescue breath should last 1 second. • Blow just enough to make the chest rise.

Continue CPR until:

1. The person begins breathing.
2. Other rescuer(s) (eg, trained first aid provider, EMS personnel) take over.
3. An AED arrives and is used. (Pause compressions to apply AED and analyze the heart rhythm, then begin compressions immediately if a shock is not advised or once a shock has been delivered as indicated by the AED.)
4. You become physically exhausted and unable to continue. (This might be prevented by having another person, if available, trade off every 5 sets of CPR [2 minutes]. Also, if you are alone, you could consider performing compression-only CPR.)

Defibrillation

If available, use an AED as soon as possible.

1. Turn on the AED.
2. Attach the pads on the person's bare, dry chest (as shown on the pads' diagrams). If needed, plug the cables into the AED. Child-sized pads may be available.
3. Stay clear of the person. Make sure no one, including you, is touching the person. Say, "Clear!"
4. Allow the AED to analyze the heart rhythm. The AED will prompt one of two actions:
   - Stay clear and press the Shock button.
   - Do not shock but give CPR, starting with chest compressions with the pads staying in place.

After performing any one of the actions, give 5 sets of CPR (2 minutes) unless the person moves, begins to breathe, or wakes up. Even if the person wakes up, leave AED pads on until EMS arrives. Repeat defibrillation Steps 3 and 4 until the person moves, begins to breathe, or wakes up; EMS arrives and takes over; or the AED states that CPR is not indicated. For an infant or small child, check to see if pediatric equipment is available. If pediatric equipment is not available, use the adult equipment. Avoid having the pads touch each other by placing one pad in the middle of the chest and the other pad on the back, between the shoulder blades.

Appendix B: Bleeding Control

Cardiopulmonary resuscitation (CPR) is designed to keep blood circulating throughout the body so that oxygen continues to be delivered to vital organs (eg, brain, heart). However, this only works if the body has sufficient blood; if a significant amount of blood is lost, less oxygen can be transported, resulting in damage to the body's tissues. For this reason, control of life-threatening bleeding must occur *before* CPR, to ensure that enough blood remains to properly oxygenate the brain and heart. CPR will be of no help if the person bleeds to death first. If two rescuers are available at an emergency scene, one should control life-threatening bleeding while the other begins CPR without delay.

The following skill sheets provide an overview of bleeding control using direct pressure (**SKILL SHEET B-1**) and a manufactured tourniquet (**SKILL SHEET B-2**).

Skill Sheet B-1 Bleeding Control

Note: Always take standard precautions.

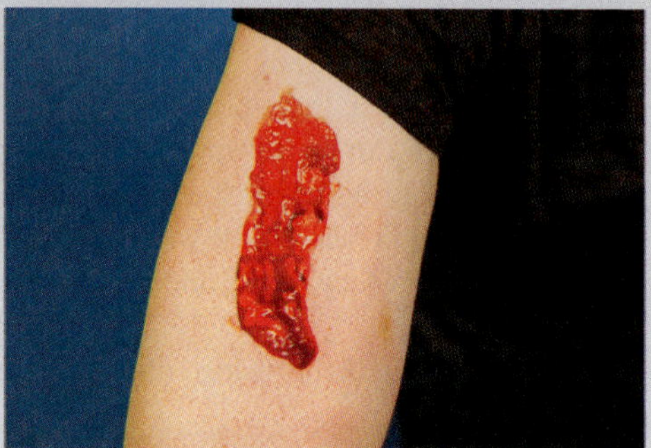

1 If the person is responsive, ask if you can help them. Expose the wound. If life-threatening bleeding is seen or suspected, call 9-1-1.

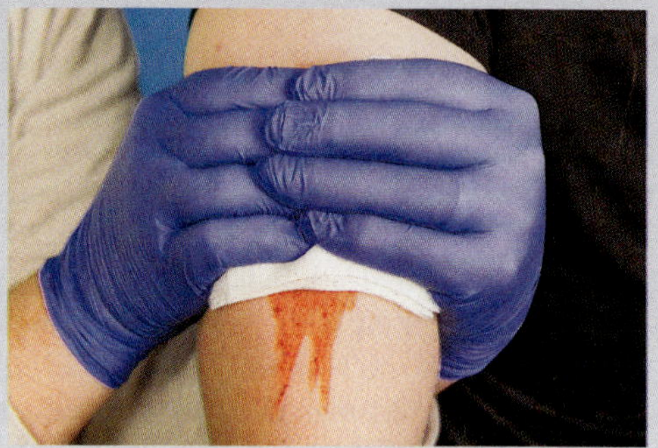

2 Cover the wound with a sterile dressing or clean cloth (eg, shirt, handkerchief, washcloth, towel). Apply firm, continuous direct pressure using the flat part of your fingers for small wounds or with the palm of your hand for large wounds. If possible, have the person apply pressure with their own hand. Keep applying pressure until the bleeding stops. If you do *not* have a sterile dressing or clean cloth, use your gloved hand. For extremities, if direct pressure does not stop life-threatening bleeding within the first minute, apply a manufactured tourniquet (see Step 5 for proper tourniquet application). **DO NOT** remove or apply any pressure on an impaled object.

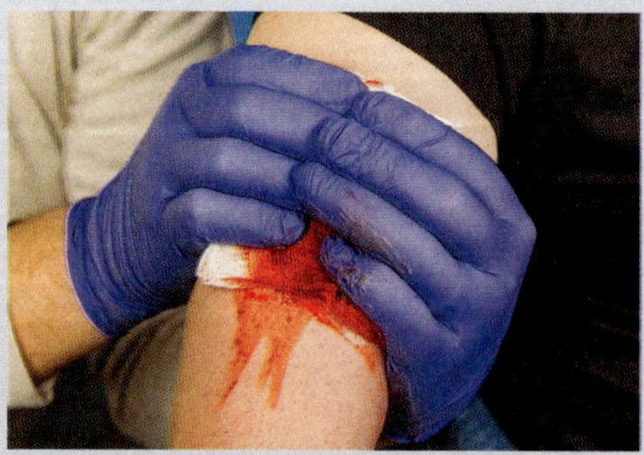

3 If a stack of dressings becomes blood-soaked, remove all but the first layer and apply better-aimed pressure using clean dressings.

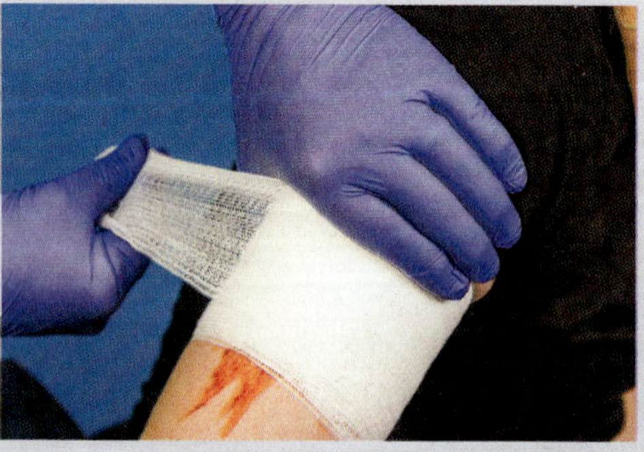

4 If direct pressure stops the bleeding, apply a pressure bandage and continue to monitor in case bleeding resumes.

Skill Sheet B-1 Bleeding Control

(continued)

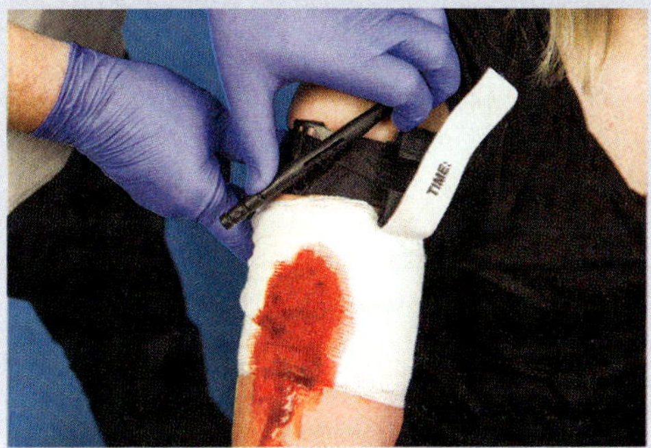

5 If direct pressure fails to immediately stop bleeding from an arm or leg, apply a manufactured tourniquet (see Skill Sheet B-2). Do not loosen or remove a tourniquet once it has been placed. For other body areas where a tourniquet placement is impossible (eg, neck, shoulders, groin) or when a tourniquet is ineffective or not available, stuff a hemostatic gauze dressing (special dressing that helps clot the blood) directly into the wound (ie, not merely applying it as a cover) until the wound is tightly packed. Apply firm, direct pressure over it for up to 10 minutes or until bleeding stops. If a hemostatic dressing is not available, stuff any gauze or clean cloth into the wound.

Consider using an improvised tourniquet if a manufactured tourniquet is not available and direct pressure or a hemostatic dressing fails to stop life-threatening bleeding.

6 After the bleeding stops, continue to monitor the injury until EMS arrives. If bleeding restarts, resume direct pressure. If bleeding resumes after a tourniquet was applied, the tourniquet is not tight enough. Tighten the tourniquet. If it is still ineffective, apply a second tourniquet near the first, above it if possible. A second tourniquet is rarely needed.

Skill Sheet B-2 Massive Bleeding Control: Applying a Manufactured Tourniquet

Apply a manufactured tourniquet to save a life when direct pressure cannot stop the bleeding (see Skill Sheet B-1, *Bleeding Control*). Remember to always take standard precautions.

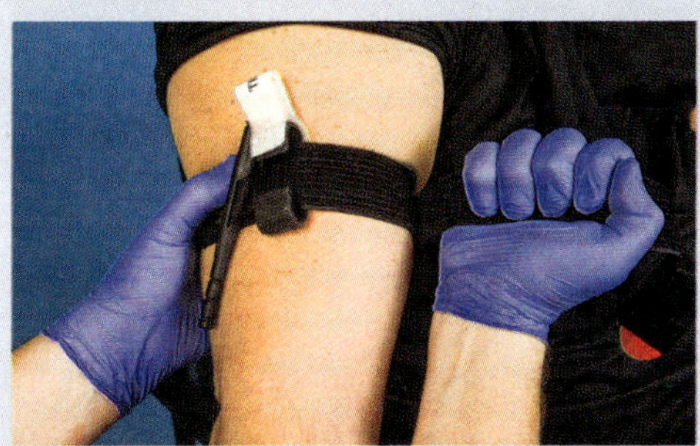

1 Ensure that 9-1-1 has been called. Quickly examine the extremity. If only one bleeding site is confirmed, place the tourniquet 2 to 3 inches (5 to 8 cm) above the wound. Otherwise, or if the size of the limb sharply tapers from large to narrow, apply the tourniquet high and tight, meaning as high on the limb as possible (see the *Tourniquet Placement box* on p. 49). When in doubt, apply it high and tight. **DO NOT** apply a tourniquet anywhere other than an arm or leg. **DO NOT** apply it over a joint (eg, elbow, wrist, knee); place it above the joint. **DO NOT** apply it over bulky clothing (eg, jackets or jeans); remove clothing before application.

(continues)

Skill Sheet B-2 Massive Bleeding Control: Applying a Manufactured Tourniquet

(continued)

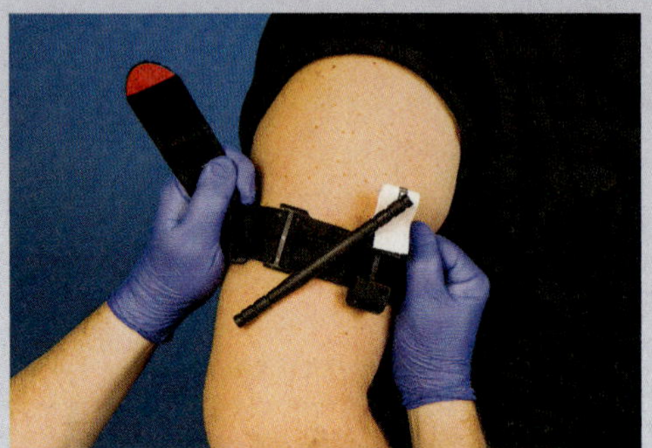

2 Tell the person that they will feel pain as you tighten the tourniquet but that it is necessary to control the bleeding. Pull the free end of the tourniquet enough to remove any slack and make it as tight as possible, then secure the free end. Thread the Velcro strap through the buckle and pull firmly on the end strap to tighten the tourniquet.

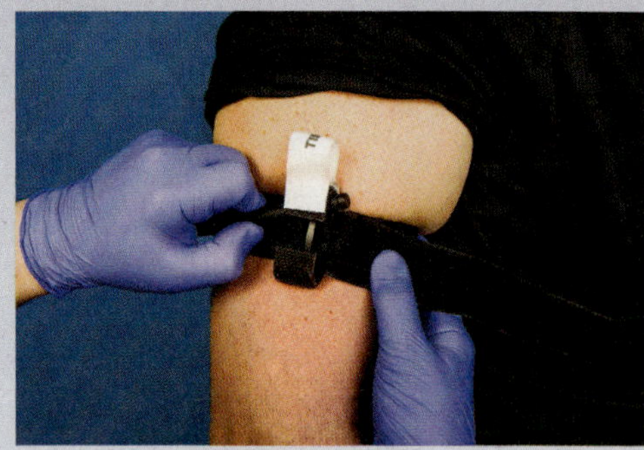

3 Continue tightening the tourniquet by twisting the rod in one direction until bleeding stops or until you can't twist it anymore. Then, secure the rod in place using the Velcro or holder to prevent it from untwisting. If the person complains of pain at any point, acknowledge it and reiterate that it is necessary to save their life or limb.

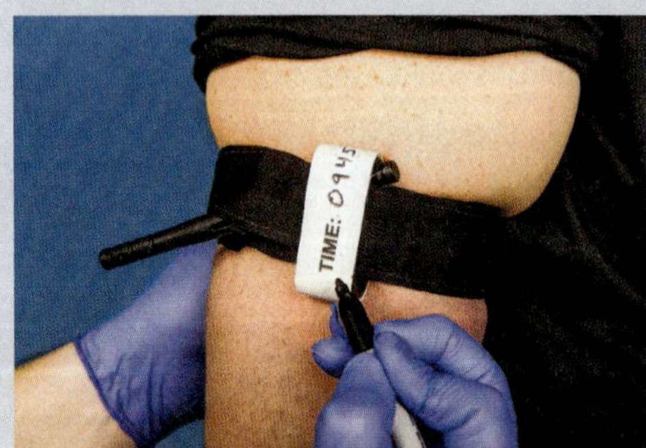

4 Write the time it was applied on the tourniquet's tag. If a tag is not available, write on a piece of tape "TQ" or "TK" for tourniquet and the time applied, and stick it on the person's forehead. **DO NOT** cover, release, or remove the tourniquet.

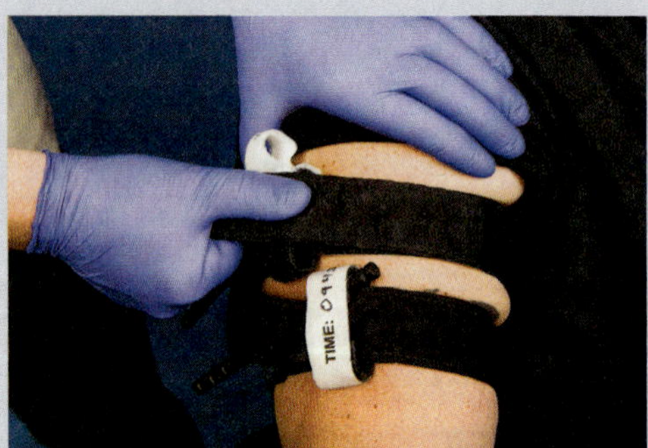

5 If life-threatening bleeding continues, the tourniquet is not tight enough. Tighten the tourniquet. If it is still ineffective, apply a second tourniquet near the first, above it if possible. A second tourniquet is rarely needed.

FYI

Tourniquet Placement

Tourniquet placement has long been a source of controversy. The two main approaches are positioning it "2 to 3 inches above the wound" or positioning it "high and tight" (meaning as high on the limb as possible, often near the armpit or groin). Place a tourniquet 2 to 3 inches above the wound when there are no active threats and the location of the wound is clear. Place a tourniquet high and tight if:

- There are active threats present.
- The wound location cannot be quickly and easily identified.
- There are multiple wounds on the limb.
- The size of the limb sharply tapers from large to narrow, such as in larger individuals.

When in doubt, place a tourniquet high and tight. Stopping life-threatening bleeding is always more important than perfect tourniquet placement.

FYI

Common Tourniquet Mistakes

- Not using a tourniquet when you should
- Using a tourniquet for minimal bleeding
- Not making the tourniquet tight enough to stop bleeding
- Using narrow material such as rope, wire, string, cord, or belt
- Waiting too long to apply the tourniquet on life-threatening bleeding
- Periodically loosening the tourniquet to allow blood flow to the injured extremity
- Not monitoring its effectiveness
- Applying over bulky clothing
- Using a tourniquet that is too large (eg, using an adult tourniquet on a child)

Index

Note: Page numbers followed by *f or t* denote figures and tables, respectively.

R

S

T

U

V

W